Complex Ethics Consultations

T0211097

Complex Ethics Consultations

Cases that Haunt Us

Edited by

Paul J. Ford and Denise M. Dudzinski

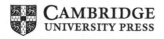

CAMBRIDGE
UNIVERSITY PRESS

CAMBRIDGE
UNIVERSITY PRESS

University Printing House, Cambridge CB2 8BS, United Kingdom

Cambridge University Press is part of the University of Cambridge.

It furthers the University's mission by disseminating knowledge in the pursuit of education, learning and research at the highest international levels of excellence.

www.cambridge.org
Information on this title: www.cambridge.org/9780521697156

First published 2008
Reprinted 2010

A catalogue record for this publication is available from the British Library

ISBN 978-0-521-69715-6 Paperback

Contents

Contributors

George J. Agich, PhD, is Director of the BGeXperience (University Values) Program and Professor of Philosophy at Bowling Green State University. His books include *Dependence and Autonomy in Old Age* (Cambridge, 2003) and his research interests include autonomy in long-term care, as well as clinical, organizational, and research ethics.

Ellen W. Bernal, PhD, is Director of Ethics at St. Vincent Mercy Medical Center in Toledo, Ohio. Her research interests include quality in end-of-life care and ethics consultation. She leads ethics education in residency programs and is a past president of the Bioethics Network of Ohio.

Mark J. Bliton, PhD, is Associate Professor of Medical Ethics and of Obstetrics and Gynecology at the Vanderbilt University School of Medicine. His areas of academic and clinical interests include the values expressed in innovative maternal–fetal surgical interventions – the focus of *Parental Voices in Maternal–Fetal Surgery,* a Symposium in the recent volume of *Clinical Obstetrics and Gynecology* (2005), which he coedited with Larry R. Churchill.

Donald Brunnquell, PhD, is Director of the Office of Ethics at Children's Hospitals and Clinics of Minnesota. His training as a child clinical psychologist informs his work in clinical ethics. He also teaches at the University of Minnesota.

Alice Chang, MSW, LICSW, is a transplant social worker at the University of Washington Medical Center. She is also a member of Ethics Consultation Service, as well as the Ethics Advisory Committee for the medical center.

Debra Craig, MD, MA, is Associate Professor of Internal Medicine at Loma Linda University. She is trained as an internist, geriatrician, and clinical ethicist. Her interest is in the ethical challenges at the end of life.

Barbara J. Daly, PhD, RN, FAAN, is Director of Clinical Ethics, University Hospitals of Cleveland, and Professor in the School of Nursing and School of Medicine, University Hospitals Case Medical Center, Cleveland, Ohio.

Joseph P. DeMarco, PhD, is Professor Emeritus of Philosophy at the Cleveland State University. His books include *A Coherence Theory in Ethics* (1994). He is coauthor of *Law & Bioethics: A Multimedia Presentation* (2007).

Douglas S. Diekema, MD, MPH, is Director of Education at the Treuman Katz Center for Pediatric Bioethics at Children's Hospital and Regional Medical Center in Seattle, Washington, where he also practices pediatric emergency medicine. He is Professor of Pediatrics at the University of Washington, with adjunct appointments in the Department of Medical History and Ethics and the School of Public Health.

Denise M. Dudzinski, PhD, MTS, is Assistant Professor in the Department of Medical History and Ethics, University of Washington School of Medicine. She is Chief of the Ethics Consultation Service, and provides organizational ethics consultation at the University of Washington Medical Center.

Stuart G. Finder, PhD, is Director of the Center for Healthcare Ethics at Cedars-Sinai Medical Center in Los Angeles. As both clinician and researcher, he is interested in exploring the complexity and implications of moral experiences as actualized in healthcare contexts.

Mary Beth Foglia, MA, RN, PhD, is Director of Preventive Ethics and a senior ethics consultant at the Veteran's Health Administration's National Center for Ethics in Health Care. Her interests include empirical ethics, ethics and quality improvement, and organizational influences on ethical healthcare practice.

Paul J. Ford, PhD, is Associate Staff, Bioethics and Neurology, at the Cleveland Clinic Foundation and Assistant Professor at Cleveland Clinic Lerner College of Medicine of Case Western Reserve University, Cleveland. His interests center on ethical issues in complex neurosurgical procedures, as well as, more broadly, on ethics consultation.

Cynthia Griggins, PhD, MA, is a neuropsychologist and ethics consultant at University Hospitals Case Medical Center and Co-Director of its Clinical Ethics Service. Her special interests include mental health and neuroethics, as well as ethics education in developing countries.

D. Micah Hester, PhD, is Associate Professor of Medical Humanities and Pediatrics at the University of Arkansas for Medical Sciences, Arkansas Children's Hospital. He has authored and edited seven books, including *Community as Healing* (2001) and *Ethics By Committee* (2008).

Albert R. Jonsen, PhD, is Professor Emeritus of Ethics in Medicine at the School of Medicine, University of Washington, and Senior Ethics Scholar in Residence at the California Pacific Medical Center, San Francisco.

Nathan A. Kottkamp, JD, is a healthcare attorney, practicing with McGuireWoods in Richmond, Virginia. He serves on several ethics committees and is the founder of the Virginia Advance Directives Day and National Healthcare Decisions Day initiatives.

Robert C. Macauley, MD, is Medical Director of Clinical Ethics at the University of Vermont College of Medicine and Fletcher Allen Health Care. Also a pediatric palliative-care physician, his research interests include end-of-life care and the influence of spirituality on clinical decision making.

Thomas R. McCormick, MDiv, DMin, is Senior Lecturer Emeritus at the University of Washington School of Medicine. His interests and research include general bioethics and transcultural issues in decision making and the care of dying patients.

Ronald B. Miller, MD, is Clinical Professor of Medicine Emeritus, at the University of California, Irvine, where he was founding Chief of the Renal Division in 1968 and founding Director of the Program in Medical Ethics in 1989. His primary interests are the ethics of nephrology, dialysis, and transplantation and of reproductive technology, stem-cell research, therapy, public policy, and end-of-life care.

Kathrin Ohnsorge, lic.Phil, MAS, is research assistent at the Unit for Ethics in Biosciences at the University of Basel, Switzerland. Her research interests are in ethics of end-of-life care, deliberative and hermeneutic approaches in bioethics, and the democratic legitimation of ethical decision making.

Robert R. Orr MD, CM, is an ethics consultant at Fletcher Allen Health Care in Burlington, Vermont, and Professor of Bioethics in the Bioethics Program, Graduate College, Union University, Schenectady, New York. He writes and teaches about the ethics consultation process and end-of-life care.

Robert A. Pearlman, MD, MPH, is Professor of Medicine at the University of Washington, Director of the Ethics Program at VA Puget Sound Health Care System, and Chief of Evaluation at the National Center for Ethics in Health Care (VHA). His interests include empirical ethics, the interplay between ethics and quality improvement, and ethical leadership.

Rosa Lynn Pinkus, PhD, is Professor of Medicine/Neurosurgery; Director, Consortium Ethics Program; and Associate Director, Center for Bioethics and Health Law, The University of Pittsburgh. Her books include (with Mark Kuczewski) *An Ethics Casebook for Hospitals: Practical Approaches to Everyday Ethics* (1999).

Joel Potash, MD, is a family physican and is Emeritus Professor at the Center for Bioethics and Humanities and Clinical Professor (voluntary) in the Department of Family Medicine, Upstate Medical University, Syracuse, New York. He is also board certified by the American Board of Hospice and Palliative Medicine.

Daryl Pullman, PhD, is Professor of Medical Ethics in the Faculty of Medicine, Memorial University, Newfoundland and Labrador, Canada. He is a member of a number of national ethics committees, including the Canadian Institutes of Health Research Standing Committee on Ethics. He has published widely in both research and clinical ethics.

Tarris D. Rosell, DMin, PhD, is Associate Professor of Pastoral Theology in Ethics and Ministry Praxis at Central Baptist Theological Seminary, and a Program

Associate at the Center for Practical Bioethics. He is a clinical ethics consultant at St. Luke's Cancer Institute and also does adjunctive bioethics instruction for William Jewell College and the Kansas City University of Medicine and Biosciences.

Sarah E. Shannon, PhD, RN, is Associate Professor in the School of Nursing and Adjunct Professor in the School of Medicine at the University of Washington, Seattle. Her research interests include end-of-life decision making with families of critically ill patients and team disclosure of errors to patients.

Rick Singleton, DMin, is Director of Pastoral Care and Ethics with Eastern Health in Newfoundland and Labrador, Canada. His interests and involvements include clinical ethics and facilitation of ethics consultations. He is Chair of Canadian Institute of Health Research Ethics Designates Caucus.

Joy D. Skeel, BSN, MDiv, is Professor in the Departments of Psychiatry and Internal Medicine, University of Toledo College of Medicine. She is Director of the Clinical Ethics Consultation Service and Director of the Ethics Program at the University of Toledo Medical Center.

Stella L. Smetanka, Esquire, is Clinical Professor of Law at the University of Pittsburgh School of Law. She directs and supervises law student practice in its Health Law Clinic through which low-income clients are afforded legal assistance related to their health care.

Jeffrey Spike, PhD, is Associate Professor of Medical Humanities and Social Sciences at the Florida State University College of Medicine. He has published 20 case studies in the *Journal of Law, Medicine, and Ethics* and the *Journal of Clinical Ethics*. His professional focus has been on defining standards for the consultation process and the proper training for consultants and on the specific competency of assessing decision-making capacity, which he believes is at the core of most ethics consults. He is member of the Editorial Board of the *American Journal of Bioethics*.

Alissa Hurwitz Swota, PhD, is Assistant Professor in the Department of Philosophy, University of North Florida. She is the Senior Fellow in Bioethics at the Blue Cross Blue Shield of Northeast Florida Center for Ethics, Public Policy, and the Professions. Her research interests include clinical ethics, cultural issues in the clinical setting, and pediatric bioethics.

Janet Templeton, BN, RN, is Regional Director of Clinical Efficiency for Eastern Health in Newfoundland and Labrador, Canada. In her role, she is responsible for patient flow and was responsible for developing and implementing the first-available-bed policy in the city hospitals.

Kathryn L. Weise, MD, MA, is a pediatric intensive care physician and ethics consultant at the Cleveland Clinic. She also serves as a member of the Cleveland Clinic Ethics Committee, Fellowship Director of the Cleveland Fellowship in Advanced Bioethics, and Director of Pediatric Palliative Care.

Kristi S. Williams, MD, is Associate Professor of Psychiatry at the University of Toledo College of Medicine. She is Director of Adult Outpatient Services and Director of the General Psychiatry Residency Program.

Gerald R. Winslow, PhD, is Professor of Ethics at Loma Linda University and Vice President for Mission and Culture at Loma Linda University Medical Center. His books include *Triage and Justice* (1982) and *Facing Limits* (1993).

David Woodrum, MD, is Professor of Pediatrics at the University of Washington School of Medicine; an ethics consultant and member of the Ethics Advisory Committee at the University of Washington Medical Center; a member of the Truman Katz Center for Pediatric Bioethics; and an ethics consultant and Chairman of the Ethics Committee at Children's Hospital and Regional Medical Center.

Richard M. Zaner, PhD, is Ann Geddes Stahlman Professor Emeritus of Medical Ethics and Philosophy of Medicine, Vanderbilt University Medical Center, Nashville, Tennessee. He currently lives in Houston, where he continues to write and present papers and narratives at various conferences. His books include *Ethics and the Clinical Encounter* (1988; 2005) and *Conversations on the Edge* (2004).

Foreword

A book on "Cases that Haunt Us" is a summons to realism in clinical ethics. Since the origins of bioethics in the 1970s, and since its turn into the clinical world in the 1980s, bioethicists have fretted over theories, principles, and methods. They have explored the theories that philosophers have created to think about and resolve ethical problems, filling pages with explanations of deontology and consequentialism. They have argued over the definitions and priorities of autonomy, beneficence, and justice. They have delved into antique methods, such as casuistry, and devised new ones, such as Rawlsian reflective equilibrium. In all of these efforts, ethics appears as a rational activity, striving to define, analyze, and resolve a problem. Certainly, some approaches, such as narrative ethics, discount the claims of excessive rationality, and casuistry disclaims the value of rational deduction. Still, bioethicists, particularly those who engage in clinical consultation, have hoped to be "solvers" of problems.

In the opening days of bioethics, one of its founders, Dan Callahan, called for the construction of a discipline that employed philosophical logic and explored "the unfettered imagination, the ability to envision alternatives, to get into people's ethical agonies . . . and sensitivity to feelings and emotions." Still, in its conclusions, bioethical thinking should reach "reasonably specific and clear decisions in the circumstances of medicine and science."[1]

"The circumstances of medicine" do present a basic problem to philosophical ethics. "Reasonably clear and specific decisions" are often confounded by the tragedies of death and disability, by the uncertainty of diagnosis and treatments, and the complexity of cases that include not only a patient and a doctor but a surrounding family, religion, money, hospital, and many other social structures. Indeed, the very notion of a "case" is perplexing. Its etymology is properly from the Latin word *casus*, which literally means "an event, an occasion." We know that any event, say a birthday party, is not simply a gathering between walls for a few hours. It radiates out into the lives of many people before and after the instant occasion. But another Latin word, *capsa*, becomes *cassa* and *caja* in the Romance languages and "case" in English. This "case" means a box or a container, as in "briefcase" or

---

1. D Callahan, *Bioethics as a Discipline*. Hastings Center Studies, 1973; 1: 66–73.

"suitcase." The coincidence of words is suggestive: bioethicists try to fit the almost infinite complications of an event into a box, where they can be studied in hopes of reaching a judgment about how they relate to each other. Of course, medicine and law do exactly the same. Their cases are defined and circumscribed sets of facts put into boxes drawn by the parameters of statutes or of pathophysiology. The process of reaching a conclusion, whether it is made by judge or physician, requires that complexity be put into order.

The clinical ethicist works with the same paradigm. However, something may be missing from that paradigm. At the heart of many ethical cases lies genuine paradox. The fine British moral philosopher, Stuart Hampshire, wrote a book titled *Morality and Conflict*. He confessed to a significant shift in his thought about morality. He once believed that "the basis of morality is found principally in powers of mind that are common to all mankind . . . improvement of human life is to come from improved reasoning . . . Slowly, I have come to disbelieve that reason, in its recognized forms, can have, and should have, that overriding role . . . I argue that morality and conflict are inseparable: conflict between different admirable ways of life and between different defensible moral ideals, conflict of obligations, conflict between essential, but incompatible interests."[2]

The ethicist is very likely to encounter conflict at the heart of a case, and the conflict is often irreconcilable. A judicial decision can slice through the conflicts of law, and physician can leap into the uncertainties of diagnosis. An ethicist may have to simply stand before irreconcilable conflict of principle. Indeed, we often speak of ethical dilemmas in which either conflicting answer to a question makes equal sense. We speak of ethical "perplexity," unconsciously evoking the ancient meaning of that word, "tangled in a net." In common conversation, people often say that moral problems are unsolvable. We ethicists may bristle at that statement because if it is true, we would seem to be superfluous. We may answer that the difficult problems are compounded of unclear thinking and missing information. We will resolve them once we resolve those issues. This answer is correct, but not always.

It does not respond to the kinds of cases reported in this book. It does not respond to the cases of conflict over "different admirable ways of life, different defensible moral ideals, conflicts of obligations, of essential but incompatible interests." It does not address the elements of consultation that the authors report in this book. These cases are filled with Hampshire's conflicts of obligations and of interests. As I read their sensitive stories and reflections, the cases of my own 30 years as a consultant floated back into my memory. Almost every case echoed in my own experience. As I now reflect on their stories and on my career as consultant, I believe that, in addition to the conflicts pointed out by Hampshire, the moral experiences encountered by ethics consultants demonstrate two ineradicable features of moral

2. S Hampshire, *Morality and Conflict*. Cambridge: Harvard University Press, 1983; p.1.

life not often discussed in moral treatises. They are the embedding of the moral problem in time and the density of the human crowd that surrounds it. The dimension of time and of a space filled with people is, I think, common to moral life in general. It is vividly present in the activities of ethics consultation in clinical medicine.

In my immature days as a scholar of ethics, ethical problems appeared in my books as timeless moments: whether or not to tell a lie, whether or not to save a threatened life. Also, these ethical problems existed in the conscience of the one who must chose, or between several persons debating right and wrong. When I entered the world of clinical medicine, ethical problems suddenly were swept into a temporal sea, moving, changing, sweeping to an ever-receding horizon. Cases concerned persons with a developing illness, an immanent crisis, a constantly shifting physiological picture, and deepening emotional responses. I was surprised by the clinicians' oft uttered phrase, "We should give this some time." For me, ethics was timelessly true.

In this book, many stories involve time. Macauley and Orr tell of a "quick" decision to withdraw life support from a neonate; Woodrum and McCormick, in contrast, are distressed by how long a case "drags out." Diekema and Spike ponder the problem of deciding prematurely or tardily. Sarah Shannon speaks of "slowing down the train" that speeds to a decision, often so fast that significant features of the case are blurred or missed. Many other chapters show the case evolving in time. Time, in medicine, may not "heal all," but certainly, it is the theater in which ethically relevant features, such as seriousness of disease, futility of treatment, hope of cure, all are played out. Bioethicists, such as those who write these chapters, have discovered that ethical problems are not static, and, much to their own moral distress, they and others often miss the opportune moment (if there is one).

The second intractable feature of moral decisions, as they appear in a clinical ethics consultation, is the density of the human crowd surrounding the patient. The ethical problem is not a proposition isolated in the mind of one or two actors – it dwells within a pressing crowd of persons, each with a distinct and rich store of interests, understandings, emotions, and personal histories. I realized, on my introduction into the world of medicine that I was no longer a priest in a confessional, which I had been for some years. The ethical experience of confession and counseling is a closed, private one. I now found myself in a hospital room, the patient in the bed, the doctors and nurses at bedside, the family waiting anxiously outside, and many other unseen participants, such as the hospital administrators, the insurers, the legal counsel, the ministers, and congregation of a church. Each of these participants views the case differently, some perhaps drastically so.

Many of the cases in this book describe the ways in which that crowd affects the consultation. Pinkus, Smetanka, and Kottkamp show a child attempting to control her treatment amid the powerful influences of family, doctors, and lawyers. Ford's patient is also caught in this crowd. Bioethicists often propose themselves as mediators and facilitators, but often, the crowd is so dense and the interests of its members so intense that mediation is futile. We try to thin out the crowd, narrow down the participants to "appropriate" ones, but sometimes fail. When some in the crowd are strangers in belief and culture to the providers and the ethicists, the negotiation becomes even more difficult. Those in the crowd may stand with banners of deeply held principles on which they will never compromise. Ohnsorge and Ford, Rosell, and Weise present versions of this story. The density of the crowd surrounding the patient puts ethics into a maelstrom of conflicting values.

These two features of moral reality make for difficult, indeed, haunting cases. They haunt in two ways. In a troubling but less profound way, they linger in the memory. We cannot get out of our heads the face of a dying child whose parents disagree over her treatment; we cannot erase the distress of an immigrant family caught in a system they do not understand. But more problematic, these hauntings are an indefinable presence dwelling in the house of bioethics. It is important for bioethicists to acknowledge that presence and to know they cannot exorcize it. It is a presence that, despite its ghostly form, puts realism into their work. They should be conscious that, often enough, they are working around, or helping others to work around, irreconcilable conflict. They should continue their task of helping unravel an ethical conflict with humility, remaining sensitive to the idea that the perplexity they encounter when they begin may still be present when they conclude their best efforts.

We modern folk, particularly those of us who revere science and scientific thinking, may be troubled by this feature of ethics. We do want to draw "reasonably specific and clear" answers out of confusing questions. We want to believe that we can devise a method of logical analysis for an ethical problem. We want the "boxes" of our cases to be uncluttered, well-sorted containers of facts and principles. Our patron philosopher, although he is unacknowledged in contemporary bioethics, may be Baruch Spinoza, who strove to create an "ethics according to geometric methods." Short of that desire for clarity, what can we ethicists do in the face of our haunting ghosts of irreconcilable conflict, the rush of time, and the density of crowds?

Professor Hampshire has a suggestion that may salve our conscience. At the end of his book, he notes that "in . . . life, the practical need is often for sensitive observation of the easily missed features of the situation, not clear application of principles . . . We have no pressing need for satisfactory total explanations of our conduct and way of life. Our need is rather to construct and maintain a way of life of which we are not ashamed and which we shall not, on reflection, regret . . . and which we respect."[3] The clinical ethicist will often observe and point out to others "the easily missed features of the situation." This is not, in the complex world of contemporary health care, a negligible contribution. In the last analysis, however,

3. Ibid., p. 168.

the ethicist, the patient, the family, the physicians, and the nurses should come away from an ethical dilemma with a resolution of which they are not ashamed, if not with "a satisfactory total explanation of conduct." They can respect the fact that thoughtful, compassionate, honest attention has been given to a deeply troubling, perplexing human problem.

The moving stories and the thoughtful reflections in this book do, as I said earlier, summon us to realism about moral life and moral decisions within medicine. Read in isolation, they may convince some that the bioethicist's life is difficult and futile. However, these authors are obviously not discouraged. They are encouraged by the resolutions that result from thoughtful, compassionate attention a case often brings. They are gratified by the relief that comes to all participants when the tension of an ethical crisis, if not extinguished, is at least relaxed by their sensitive, wise involvement.

Fortunately, ethics is not, as Pullman, Singleton, and Templeton note in their concluding chapter, all hard cases. It is an amalgam of centuries of thought about the moral life of humans, broadly accepted moral principles of modern bioethics, and the collections of many cases. The "hard cases" appear within that broader perspective. The emotional discomfort and the intellectual puzzlement of these cases do not undermine the experience of respect, beneficence, compassion, and justice that bioethicists and, indeed, all providers of care can view as a guide to their professional endeavors. In this way, "respect," not "regret," will mark the life and work of this new profession.

Albert R. Jonsen
Professor Emeritus of Ethics in Medicine
School of Medicine, University of Washington

Senior Ethics Scholar in Residence
California Pacific Medical Center
San Francisco, California

Acknowledgments

The idea for this book arose during a dinner with our mentor Richard Zaner at a conference. We identified the need for sharing cases that emphasize the affective component of ethics consultation. Richard Zaner's influence can be seen throughout many aspects of this work, and we are greatly indebted to him. That conversation prompted us to present several panels discussing haunting cases and to edit a special section of the *Journal of Clinical Ethics (JCE)*. We continue to be grateful to those at *JCE* who fostered the publication of the original cases that are included, with revision, in this book. We are especially grateful to Norman Quist, Randy Howe, Mary Gesford, and Leslie LeBlanc. We would like to thank those at Cambridge University Press who believed deeply in the text as this project transformed into a book. They include Richard Barling, Pauline Graham, and Rachael Lazenby and, more recently, Nicholas Dunton and Katie James.

Denise is indebted to Paul Ford, who is a first-rate collaborator and whose talent, hard work, and humility make him a pleasure to work with. She is especially grateful to her husband, Michael Fanning, for his unwavering support, encouragement, patience, and the happiness he brings her. Her son, Max, brings her joy and pride and energized her work on the book. Her parents, Mary Ann and Arthur Dudzinski have nurtured her and her career ever since she took her mom's advice to take a philosophy course. Her sister, Katie McWeeny, and her family brought humor and respite in the midst of the book preparation. Mark Bliton, Stuart Finder, Kate Payne, and John Johnson advised and encouraged her during her training and provided incredible opportunities to teach and to learn about ethics consultation. She is also indebted to staff and faculty in the Department of Medical History and Ethics at the University of Washington.

Paul thanks Denise Dudzinski, who brought compassion, patience, and keen thinking without which completion and quality would have been uncertain for this project. He would especially like to thank Gwen and Gary Ford for their generous support throughout his career and education. They instilled a strong sense of pragmatism and compassion that serves him well. His wife, Laura McMullen Ford, has been patient and supportive at each turn and provided many helpful comments during the most difficult moments. His daughter, Meredith Mackenzie Ford, was a strong source of encouragement and strength during the final year of development.

On an academic side, John Lachs and Keith Johnson provided opportunities and mentoring that continue to be influential. George Agich apprenticed Paul in ethics consultation with special emphases on careful listening and constant openness to interpretation. Finally, the many colleagues at the Cleveland Clinic deserve his deepest gratitude for their collaborative spirit.

In particular, we would like to thank Mary Adams and Jennifer Cook for helping with the finally editing and organization of these chapters. Many people whom we have not mentioned explicitly have commented and provided administrative support. We also appreciate their efforts.

Finally, we would like to acknowledge all of the patients, families, and healthcare providers who have had faith in the services of ethics consultants. We and our colleagues carry a significant responsibility when people place faith in us.

Live and learn: courage, honesty, and vulnerability

Paul J. Ford and Denise M. Dudzinski

Introductory comments

The cases in this volume exemplify a rich cross-section of consultation experiences from which we can learn. The authors tell stories and share personal responses connected to deeply affective clinical ethics cases in which they consulted. None of these authors has selected an easy case. Ambiguity, second-guessing, and regret permeate their stories and reflections. They show great courage in laying bare such things as potential missteps, institutional impotence, and interpersonal struggles. Through their openness, we have amassed a rare collection of stories from which to learn about real-life challenges encountered by clinical ethics consultants in the incredibly complex world of contemporary health care.

Although overarching themes emerge in this volume, these cases should be read with an open mind since these themes may not be those stereotypically found in bioethics textbooks. Our cases identify challenges including uncertainty about decision-making capacity, limiting treatment requests, and obligations of health-care providers to protect patients. The cases go beyond just tragedy. They touch on uncertainty, lack of power, and unclear professional boundaries that blend to create a mix of end-of-life, quality-of-life, organizational, and societal concerns. Naturally, the end-of-life cases represent a significant portion of this volume given the high stakes. In these end-of-life cases the endorsement of withdrawal of therapy comes alternately from families and healthcare providers. As we see from experience, the role played in a case, whether patient, family member, physician, nurse, or ethicist, does not always predict the source of a therapy-withdrawal request. Clinical ethicists neither uniformly support withdrawal of therapy nor always agree with the physician's opinion. We have purposely included cases that go beyond this stereotype since troubling cases occur in outpatient practice, institutional policy

Sections adapted from Ford PJ, Dudzinski DM. Specters, Traces, and Regret in Ethics Consultation. *Journal of Clinical Ethics*, 2005; 16(3): 193–5. ©2005 by *The Journal of Clinical Ethics*. Used with permission. All rights reserved.

discussions, quality-of-life interventions, and when considering clinical innovations. The cases in this volume cover a broad range encountered in a variety of healthcare settings. In the final chapter of this book we provide guidance as to how these cases may be used in education. Below we provide general thoughts, discussions of cases, and review of selected themes to provide a richer context for reflecting on the cases.

Specters, traces, and regret

Clinical ethics consultants inevitably engage in cases that haunt them long after a formal involvement ends. As with patients, families, and care providers, ethics consultants remain moral agents with culpability for their interactions and recommendations. When consulting, ethics consultants necessarily weave themselves into the story of the case. In doing so, they influence the path of these stories, and they themselves are altered by those encounters. Standard ways of writing ethics cases focus on particular ethical issues rather than the role of, and affective impact on, the ethics consultant. Case analyses must blend substantive ethical issues with personal challenges consultants experience to get the full effect of the complexity of clinical ethics consultation. At times no good solution to a dilemma exists, organizational or legal constraints seem insurmountable, and/or the consultant is unable to bring about a result. Although ethical dilemmas should be discussed for the sake of the dilemmas themselves, sharing the affective nature of complex situations plays an important role in a consultant's professional development. By acting with integrity ethics consultants recognize their shortcomings and improve practices. Having the courage to write about these cases helps others in the field recognize the personal and professional risks of ethics consultation. Sharing haunting cases may improve the practice of clinical ethics consultation by addressing the character and professional development of consultants. Sharing these stories with clinicians and patients improves understanding of good processes needed in our current healthcare settings.

Clinical ethics consultation can be haunting for several reasons. First, there is the challenge of ethical issues themselves, which can be stressful when helping others negotiate a resolution. These elements create tense environments in which the stakes can be high. Second, a clinical ethics consultant's judgment as to when and how to intervene in a particular case influences the processes within clinical care. The involvement is not always beneficial and may occasionally cause harm. Third, consultants experience moral distress and uncertainty similar to the distress and uncertainty experienced by those being helped. Fourth, consultants often feel powerless to facilitate positive change when tragedy and suffering are pervasive or organizational constraints seem intractable. Finally, once consultation commences, our values become part of the complex dynamics, either incorporated constructively or stumbled over on the road to clarity. These elements blend to create consultation experiences that long influence and affect us.

Clinical ethics consultants influence cases, if in no other way than by bringing greater understanding of individual and professional values, thereby fostering decision making. While they may encourage others to courageously express and negotiate values, consultants also risk harming others and being harmed themselves (Bliton & Finder, 2002, 233–58; Zaner, 1996, 255–77). To do consultation well, consultants need to empathize with other participants to fully appreciate the circumstances. This empathy is balanced by careful reasoning and reflection in order to influence a case to the best ends possible. To be effective, consultants invest themselves in the devastating circumstances of others and attempt to assuage suffering by facilitating critical reflection. Emotions and facts are important to the dynamics of ethics consultation. The balance of the cognitive and the emotional often manifests itself in the terms "subjective" and "objective." This is seen in a number of cases in the text, such as those contributed by Swota and by Woodrum and McCormick. Losing some "objectivity" is not necessarily negative. The subjective will not necessarily mislead the consultant if it is balanced by clear articulation and understanding of the reasons and context of the case. Consultants can positively influence circumstances by integrating experiential and analytic elements.

Hauntings must not paralyze consultants, as might be a natural response to being emotionally overwhelmed. To communicate effectively often requires recognizing the ambiguity, sorrow, uncertainty, and lack of closure inherent in many consultations. For instance, Macauley and Orr articulate a warning against being "driven to incapacitating doubt" that is echoed through numerous cases (Macauley & Orr, p. 18). Paradoxically, being haunted can also foster further professional growth and reflection that prompts increased activity. To whatever degree these special cases influence our activities by means of paralysis, growth, or anxiety, it is clear that they contain significant affective components. They influence consultants beyond their professional activities. Grief and sadness borne of tragic and frustrating cases may linger when returning to families and social circles. Given the small community of bioethicists in any given geographic area, isolation may preclude confidential debriefing, thereby confounding attempts to process these emotions. Sharing, reading, and discussing cases may decrease the sense of isolation and demonstrate that consultants are not, in fact, alone in coping with the emotional "baggage" of their work. We hope this book will provide support and facilitate open discussion.

Sections, divisions, and organization

The cases in each section are grouped by theme for certain educational purposes. However, given the depth of challenges in each case, many cases have multiple themes so that alternative ways of organizing are just as plausible. With that in mind, in the final chapter we suggest several ways to reorganize and outline teaching, discussion, and professional growth uses. Below we provide an overview of each book section.

The first section, *Starting at the beginning: prenatal and neonatal issues*, focuses on prenatal and neonatal issues. The four cases could be interpreted as pairs of cases addressing similar problems. Robert Macauley and Robert Orr's discussion of an end-of-life decision in the neonatal intensive care unit contrasts with David Woodrum and Thomas McCormick's case. Macauley and Orr discuss withdrawal of therapy on a neonate that seemed to have been accelerated over a weekend. The process of deciding is quick and did not give many on the primary team or other family members knowledge of the imminent event. Of particular note in this case is the commitment to quality improvement premised on the existence of discernible ethics consultative errors or less effective ways of doing consultation. However, the critique is tempered by the understanding that any retrospective analysis of a particular situation relies on reports rather than direct experience. The quality of ethics consultation should not be based on a bad medical outcome or on information not reasonably available at the time of the consultation. Ethics consultation is imprecise and is undertaken in the face of uncertainty. Retrospective review and criticism should be based on the information and opportunities reasonably available during the moment of decision making.

In a neonatal case where withdrawal of aggressive therapy is recommended by the medical team, Woodrum and McCormick reflect on how long the case drags out. The team anguishes while watching the baby suffer and the recommendation for withdrawal is not accepted. How should law and ethics interface in solving cases? The authors propose a legal resolution to protect the baby from undue suffering. However, in the end they believe appealing to the law may be a futile endeavor. This case provides a nice counterpoint to the first case, in which the process of deciding went very quickly.

The second two cases in this section relate to perinatal issues. Richard Zaner describes parents faced with a complicated pregnancy for which there is a great deal of prognostic uncertainty. The 22-week fetus might have spina bifida, suggested by ultrasound and alpha-feto protein tests. In speaking with the patient, Zaner discovers a subtle source of distress. The patient is astounded that such a profound decision must be made quickly, before the age of viability and without adequate clinical information. Zaner attempts to help the parents make critical treatment decisions in the midst of excruciating medical and moral uncertainty. Zaner reflects on the familiar haunting of moral decision making when the possibility for a devastating "mistake" is immense and the patient's vulnerability is great.

Mark Bliton reflects on the decision of a woman to undergo innovative maternal–fetal surgery to repair a neural-tube defect. Similar to Zaner, this story centers on a pregnant woman faced with an intractably difficult decision laden with uncertainty. In conversation with the patient, Bliton attempts to be sensitive to a suffering woman facing potentially tragic outcomes while also encouraging exploration of hidden ambiguities and value questions that she may be avoiding. Bliton's uncomfortable conversations before and after the fetal intervention prompt him to reassess consultation processes and his own values. In many ways, the uncomfortable conversations described by Bliton and Zaner challenge our underlying value assumptions. These hauntings, bred of uncertainty and lack of information, strike at the very foundation of clinical ethics consultation.

In the second section, *The most vulnerable of us: pediatrics*, cases divide evenly between inpatient and outpatient concerns. Douglas Diekema and Jeffrey Spike highlight the way cases unfold differently when physicians believe it to be premature to withdraw life-sustaining therapy and when they believe withdrawal has been delayed too long. These cases also reflect the dual roles that consultants play, with Diekema being a physician who treated the patient but subsequently acts as an ethics consultant and Spike being a nonphysician who is unexpectedly thrust into a communication role he believes should be undertaken by a physician. In Diekema's case, he treats a young girl in the emergency room who is then admitted to the intensive-care unit. His subsequent ethics consultation is further textured by the resonance he feels with the family's religious tradition. He discusses the relevance of his relationship as provider and of his sympathy and understanding of the family's religious perspective toward his ethics recommendations.

Spike describes an ethics consult called by providers who believe life-sustaining therapy should be withdrawn. The baby has sustained severe traumatic neurological damage for which the mother is criminally charged. Spike reflects on how he, as the consultant, is forced to balance a number of competing visceral reactions to an incarcerated mother who comes to her baby's bedside in chains. Is the mother who allegedly hurt the baby entitled to see her? What role should the consultant play when the physician leaves the "family" meeting to the ethics consultant? In both Spike and Diekema's cases, the consultant resists being persuaded by simple consensus but is sympathetic to the clinicians' commitment to protect a vulnerable child.

Two narratives describe complex pediatric cases where patient care occurs outside a hospital setting. Rosa Lynn Pinkus, Stella Smetanka, and Nathan Kottkamp describe a child who refuses additional chemotherapy after her cancer returns. A complex dynamic emerges among the physicians, family, lawyers at a university law clinic, and the clinical ethicist. They explore the role of the ethics consultant as a mediator, patient advocate, or consultant. Most strikingly they highlight a broken therapeutic trust and a young girl trapped by the conflict. The patient and her family select an option offered by the physicians not to undergo another round of chemotherapy. Only after they choose this option are they informed that the physician never considered it a genuine option. The family experiences this as a "bait and switch," having been told they had a choice while the medical team was only really willing to allow one of the options. Providers may believe they are adhering to standards of "informed consent" by including options they do not recommend or are unwilling to provide. Although undertaken with good intentions, this can be devastating to the therapeutic relationship.

In Micah Hester's account, the patient has a chronic need for a ventilator and is unable to participate in the decision-making process. The issues center on children who rely on medical technology in both inpatient and outpatient settings. The physicians advocate for "comfort care only" while the parents strongly prefer that the child be cared for at home and continue with intensive medical support. Hester reflects on the lack of definition of his role and regrets that he did not meet directly with the parents. Hester discusses the difficult interface between inpatient and outpatient medical care.

In the third section, *Diversity of desires and limits of liberty: psychiatric/psychological issues,* cases center on patients with psychiatric issues or mental status alterations and highlight that patients and professionals may have radically different notions of "beneficial" treatment goals. In the chapter by Joy Skeel and Kristi Williams, the patient continually makes self-destructive choices that alienate him from his care providers. During episodes of multiple readmissions, the patient has been labeled as "hateful." The consultant finds herself mediating between the individual medical services such as medicine, psychiatry, and nursing. Further, she attempts to mediate between the healthcare providers and the patient. The case raises questions about the ethics consultant's power to help and perhaps prompts regret that a more effective approach might have been missed.

Barbara Daly and Cynthia Griggins describe a patient who espouses mutually exclusive desires and goals. He has quadriplegia and does not want to be turned for decubitus wound care but also does not want to die from the sepsis that recurs because of poor wound care. In the end, the authors recommend a "Ulysses contract," which overrides the patient's decision to decline dressing changes when wound care is initiated but provides the patient with the power to dictate the timing of the care. Weekly they negotiate this agreement with the patient at which time he can decline the contract and transition to comfort care only. The authors underscore the power imbalances for disabled patients who are profoundly dependent on medical staff and who also lack family or other advocates. In reflecting on the role of the consultant, the authors ponder whether they should be negotiators or advocates. They also recognize that unlike the nursing staff, they do not have to experience the patient's protests when the contract is being enforced. They are insulated from the anguish of implementing their recommendations.

Paul Ford describes a patient with limited and sporadic cognitive function whose designated decision makers are at odds with the medical team. There is disagreement as to what would be best for the patient and what would be acceptable medical practice. The clotting off of a dialysis catheter sparks a futility discussion. Ford feels trapped in an institutional process designed to protect the disparate interests of patients, physicians, and the institution, but the process is neither expedient nor smooth in reaching a satisfactory conclusion in this case. The case questions the reactive nature of consultation and the need to occasionally deviate from policies that exact a heavy cost to all parties.

Debra Craig and Gerald Winslow describe a woman refusing to eat, which the family accepts after a while. Craig and Winslow use this case to explore the complexities of being a physician ethics consultant and to reflect on alternative approaches to consultation. The patient is discharged in the care of the husband and receives hospice nursing even though a terminal diagnosis was never found. The retrospective review of the case by the ethics committee provides a reminder of the importance of quality improvement. This reflection on peer review resonates with the earlier discussion by Macauley and Orr.

The fourth section, *Withholding therapy with a twist*, addresses the traditional question of withdrawing life-sustaining therapy; except these cases all have unusual or unexpected features. Ellen Bernal begins the section attentive to process and role. Reflecting on an experience from early in her career, she describes a woman in a Catholic hospital who consistently requests discontinuation of therapy. However, both her physician and her husband will not allow her wishes to be fulfilled. She relies on secondhand and thirdhand reports about patient wishes while the patient continues to be awake and communicating. She looks to the attending physician for "permission" to be involved. Like Ford, she reflects on the constraints of following institutional processes too rigidly. Finally, she emotionally describes the level of responsibility a clinical ethicist should assume for patient outcomes and the potential cost to interprofessional relationships. Expectations of responsibility are generated by both the ethics consultant as well as those who request the consultation. A failure of those expectations can exact a significant personal and interpersonal cost. Bernal frankly articulates how, given her current experience, she would have handled the case differently.

Joseph DeMarco and Paul Ford describe a case where a family requests withdrawal relatively soon after surgery. DeMarco provides the perspective of an academic bioethicist in his initial introduction to the world of bedside clinical ethics consultation. He observes the surgeon's mild resistance to ethics involvement, stemming from the surgeon's belief that he knows how his patient's care will proceed. The surgeon's stance changes dramatically by the end of the case, when he looks to the consultants for resolution, or absolution, after conceding that withdrawal of therapy could be enacted. It may have been the consultants' lack of verbal support for the surgeon during the family meeting that led him to agree to withdraw therapy. A consultant's aptly chosen silences in a family meeting can sometimes have as much effect as speaking volumes.

George Agich warns against blindly trusting reports about the medical facts of a case and advises consultants to avoid being used as a perfunctory ethical validation for a preconceived course of action. He discusses ventilator withdrawal with a patient and suspects the patient needs further clinical clarification of treatment options. The patient confuses the burdens of a tracheostomy in general with those she experiences because of the size of the tube. Agich demonstrates his listening acumen, which is informed by his philosophical training and his long experience as a clinical ethicist. He was able to discern essential gaps in communication. He demonstrates challenges commonly faced by nonclinician ethics consultants, such as acquiring basic knowledge of clinical facts and being familiar with the clinical context. Agich acknowledges but disputes the common perception that clinical ethicists support a "culture of death" by favoring withdrawal.

In Stuart Finder's case, he wonders why a broken jaw precipitates withdrawal of life-sustaining treatment. After exploring various perspectives, the rationale becomes clear. However, a weekend call from an administrator prompts him to second-guess whether further follow-up should have been undertaken before "signing off" on the case. Finder raises questions of how far cases should be pursued and when the consultation is closed. It can be tempting to judge a case to be complete when plans of care resonate with the consultant's personal values. In the end, the question of the influence and responsibility of the ethics consultant's actions must be recognized.

The sixth section, *The unspeakable/unassailable: religious and cultural beliefs*, addresses cases that involve cultural and religious influences on belief systems. Donald Brunnquell begins this section with a striking case of an adolescent with an ectopic pregnancy. He raises questions about confidentiality, coercion, and honesty in exploring how to respond to a young girl who could become a cultural outcast if her tight-knit community discovers her sexual activity. Is threatening the girl with police involvement if she neglects medical follow-up justified if her mother is not going to be told? Should the ethicist condone lying to the mother? Balancing the social values with the physical well-being of an adolescent becomes difficult in a cross-cultural setting. The consultant's limited access to cultural information interjects significant uncertainty.

Tarris Rosell explores living unrelated kidney donation. Religion factors into the donor's motivation to put herself at risk for a fellow member of the congregation with whom she is not well acquainted. In transplantation, ethics consultants are often asked to explore motivation, reasons, and potential coercion. Rosell explores the challenges arising from the donor's being "directed by God" to donate, the lack of an emotional connection with the recipient, and the potential for secondary gain. He also reflects on the appropriateness of recommending counseling and the apparent disregard for the consultant's recommendations. As other authors in this volume have noted, consultants must be cognizant of the burden imposed when counseling is recommended or mandated by the ethics consultant.

Physician-ethicist Kathryn Weise helps to resolve a conflict by developing and arranging an alternative-care plan while acting as an ethics consultant. She arranges for a hospice to accept a patient on a ventilator with an agreement that the ventilator will be withdrawn soon after arrival. This appears to respect a variety of the participant's desires and values. Not only does she reflect on the family's Islamic beliefs concerning medical care but also on the appropriateness of the bioethicist in coordinating discharge and being responsible for creative care solutions. Regarding the twist at the end of the case, she wonders whether she ignored her training and obligations as a physician while assuming the role of an ethicist. Perhaps by insisting on explicit consideration of stressful ethical and treatment issues, she contributed to the tangible harm that the patient's mother experiences.

Kathrin Ohnsorge and Paul Ford describe a patient who relies on a direct communication from God to make his healthcare decisions. They analyze both the hermeneutics of the case as well as the degree to which the consultant's use of religious language can be deceptive and manipulative. Finding a balance between a consultant's knowing about religious traditions, calling on those who are expert in spiritual matters, and leaving spiritual discussions to others can be very challenging. Consultants should strive for transparency, avoid manipulation of patients, and exemplify respect for patient beliefs. Also, the authors consider the possibility that a student-teacher dynamic could have influenced the consultation. Just as in medicine, we should not minimize or dismiss that trainer-trainee relationships may potentially confound the consultation.

The sixth section, *Human guinea pigs and miracles: clinical innovation/ unorthodox treatment*, involves variations in clinical practice that raise difficult issues. Denise Dudzinski recounts the story of a woman requesting the amputation of her arm because of complex regional pain syndrome. Dudzinski reflects on the moral distress she encounters and its impact on professional integrity. She contemplates when an ethics consultation is appropriate and how the consultant's own interests play into the decision for informal consultation. The case prompts consideration of professional boundaries and integrity as well as the limits to a patient's right to request unusual treatments. As well, Dudzinski takes the opportunity to speak directly with the patient even though she is not formally consulted in the case. This creates an interesting contrast to the cases where consultants do not have the opportunity to speak with patients even formally consulted.

Alissa Swota describes a case from her ethics fellowship in which there are two surrogates of equal standing. She notes the challenges in moving from being a supervised student to an independent ethics consultant. A family member demands, over the objections of his sister, that herbal remedies be used instead of standard pain medications in palliative treatment of their dying father. Throughout the case Swota weaves themes of conflict, limits of choice, and the ethics consultant's proper role. Often consultants are thrown in the midst of long-standing social and family dynamics that are impossible to solve in the brief time of ethics consultation interaction. The consultant recommends psychological counseling for the surrogates in order to improve decision-making dynamics. This pushes the boundaries of the ethics consultant's role.

Alice Chang and Denise Dudzinski tell the sad story of a patient who is tethered to a heart device designed to be a bridge to transplantation. The team struggles with the permissibility of turning off a heart device that will result in the patient's certain and quick demise. The consultants find that guidelines designed for just such a case were not helpful. In the end, this case is both rich in questions of innovative therapy and institutional ethics. As in Skeel and Williams' case, the hospital seemed to be the only "safe place" for the patient. One consultant describes feeling "all alone" in trying to discharge her duties both as a social worker and as a consultant, which raises again the dual-role challenges faced by many consultants.

Ronald Miller provides a historical perspective on altruistic living kidney donation in his discussion of the earliest debates about organ donors. While Rosell discusses a contemporary case occurring after better acceptance of living unrelated donation, Miller's case occurs just prior to this broader acceptance. Miller challenges his colleagues' skepticism about altruistic donation and their insistence on a psychiatric evaluation as mandatory for every potential altruistic donor. He believes the ethics committee should not unnecessarily require potential donors to undergo psychiatric evaluations. In Miller's story, there were no medical indications for a psychiatric evaluation other than some committee members' suspicions about her motivation for altruistic donation. Related to motivation, Miller posits that media should not be involved in order to eliminate publicity seekers. Most importantly, Miller warns again of committees entering into a kind of "group think" that becomes unreflective. Each member of a committee and consultative teams should independently consider the facts of each case in order to make a well-informed judgment.

The final section, *The big picture: organizational issues*, addresses the institutional and organizational ethics issues arising from ethical challenges in clinical cases. Although this aspect of clinical ethics consultation garners little attention, it is becoming increasingly important (Burns, 2000). Mary Beth Foglia and Robert Pearlman address the thorny issue of the responsibility institutions have for their residents' moonlighting at other hospitals. Through a complex set of events, a moonlighting resident makes an error in follow-up at an outside hospital resulting later in the death of a patient at the ethics committee's own hospital. Even when cases are formally outside the ethics committee's realm, does the committee have obligations to bring these to the attention of other hospitals, the families of patients, or the state medical board? Not to act on such information is a moral act in itself. The very knowledge of a situation may entail a moral obligation to act, particularly if an error is unlikely to be identified or disclosed without the committee's involvement. The authors explicitly raise the concept of moral error as well as the distinction between legal and moral accountability.

In some ways Joel Potash builds on the theme of error disclosure raised by Foglia and Pearlman. He articulates the ethical reasoning underpinning the recommendation to disclose a patient's possible exposure to Creutzfeldt-Jakob disease through improperly sterilized surgical instruments. The ethics committee's power may be limited in various ways, ranging from medical record access, to charting recommendations, to communicating with the patient. Although the committee acts as a consultative body, it also is called on by outside groups to play a role in creating policy and may be seen as having a duty to assure ethical practice. In the short term, the neurosurgeon does not inform the patient even though the ethics committee strongly recommends disclosure. Potash expounds on the need to publish these cases to refine our further thinking on such matters.

Sarah Shannon's narrative describes poor communication, misunderstandings, and the long delay in an ethics committee response. Bedside nurses are frustrated that a patient is pushed out of the hospital under false pretenses likely resulting in his premature death. She describes the proper roles of an ethics committee, including "slowing down the train" so that better decisions can be made, healing emotional wounds, and providing solace during retrospective reviews. She maintains that even in the retrospective review, there are important healing functions as well as opportunities to prospectively improve process. The dearth of nursing home beds as well as financial constraints act as catalysts for the sequence of tragic events in this case. As a result, the family feels pressured. Shannon confesses that teaching this case has been cathartic and helps her cope with the haunting she still experiences.

Daryl Pullman, Rick Singleton, and Janet Templeton begin the final chapter with one of the catalysts described in Shannon's chapter: the limited number of beds in skilled facilities. They explore the way in which a general policy to more efficiently allocate beds shifts costs from one population to another. Such policies should be responsive to the unusual case but rigid enough to be effective for commonly occurring cases. The individual ethics consultant should balance the ramifications of the particular case with the broader impact on patient populations. Single ethics consultations should not drive all policy. When policy is applied it should be done so respecting the underlying ethos of the relevant policies. The explicit point that policy should be based on standard circumstances rather than extraordinary ones creates an opening for re-evaluation of every single case in our book. Tough cases may cause more careful reflection on underlying assumptions, but they also should not disproportionately influence the practice of ethics consultation. Consultative methods should be based on good process that is not derailed by a single bad outcome or a particularly sad case. As in Pullman et al.'s reflection, a tough case may cause us to re-evaluate our process while still keeping our focus on ways of consultation that can be applied most broadly.

Final reflections and observations

Haunting cases are not unique to ethics consultation. These cases exist in many areas of medicine. In particular, they are common with surgical interventions. In patient management meetings where candidacy of surgery may be discussed, it is not uncommon to hear people say things like "This case looks like another Mr. Smith . . . none of us want that" or "Remember Mrs. Jones. We still don't know why surgery failed to work." These anecdotes are cautionary and indicative of the emotional affects on care providers by outcomes and processes. They are not simply, "Remember that a particular type of procedure failed." They are also about an inchoate experience that remains mysterious, anguishing, or puzzling. The cases in this text describe challenges in systems, practice, and personal involvement that haunt clinical ethics consultants.

The contributing authors represent diverse backgrounds, experiences, and styles of consultation. Their professional backgrounds include medicine, nursing, philosophy, law, psychology, social work, and religion/theology. The authors draw from a range of career development stages, which prompts reflection from students to retired consultants. Sometimes the more senior consultants choose to reflect on cases early in their consultation experiences while others reflect on more recent cases. In the cases from early in their careers there is a recurrent theme of the dynamics of being new to a profession, being new to an institution, or training issues. Cases in this volume represent individual, small group, and full committee consultation styles with many variations on the implementation of these approaches. Independent of the reader's style and background, each story resonates on a deeply personal and human level.

The case descriptions are not as comprehensive and detailed as some are accustomed to reading. However, essential clinical details are included in broad strokes. Each author has modified the case in some way, changing or leaving out details, to preserve patient and family anonymity. However, the most important part of these cases, personal and professional reflection, is not altered. Though brief, each telling of the consultation contains a rich array of ethical, professional, and emotional themes. Each chapter uniformly contains the following sections: case narrative; professional reflections/lessons; haunting issues; outcome; and discussion questions. The cases are purposely kept succinct and brief to highlight the most compelling experiences as well as to be most useful for a discussion session or an educational portion of an ethics committee meeting. We hope that these cases will be used in a variety of teaching and learning environments. The cases should not be read as endorsing any explicit method or particular judgment made by ethics consultants. However, we endorse the honesty and courage of the authors and express appreciation for all of the patients, healthcare providers, and families who invite us into their lives.

REFERENCES

Bliton MJ, Finder SG. Traversing boundaries: Clinical ethics, moral experience, and the withdrawal of life supports. *Theor Med*, 2002; 23: 233–58.

Burns JP. From case to policy: Institutional ethics at a children's hospital. *J Clin Ethics*, 2000; 11(2): 175–81.

Zaner RM. Listening or telling? Thoughts on responsibility in clinical ethics consultation. *Theor Med*, 1996; 17(3): 255–77.

Part I

Starting at the beginning: prenatal and neonatal issues

Quality of life – and of ethics consultation – in the NICU

Robert C. Macauley and Robert D. Orr

Case narrative

One Sunday afternoon, the on-call ethicist (one of the co-authors) received a consultation request from the Neonatal Intensive Care Unit (NICU) of our 500-bed academic medical center. Two weeks earlier, a baby had been born at term with skeletal, renal, cardiac, and (most profoundly) pulmonary abnormalities but no known neurologic defects. The baby had been intubated in the delivery room and subsequently developed pulmonary hypertension, requiring high ventilator settings and inspired oxygen concentration and necessitating that the patient be chemically paralyzed.

Because the patient's abnormalities were not consistent with any defined syndrome, his long-term prognosis remained unclear – the neonatology team covering on the weekend described it as "quite bleak." It was possible that the patient could become permanently ventilator-dependent, although it was also possible that he would eventually breathe on his own, albeit still with limb deformities and renal problems. The only certainty at that time was that the patient would require weeks to months of ventilatory support to survive.

Two days earlier, the NICU team had met with the family, and the decision was made to de-escalate the patient's level of life support by withdrawing chemical paralysis and making the patient DNR (do not resuscitate). Although mechanical ventilation was continued, most people involved in the case (including the patient's parents) did not expect the baby to survive. However, to everyone's surprise, over the next 48 hours, his respiratory condition stabilized and even improved. On Sunday afternoon, the parents requested discontinuation of mechanical ventilation.

The covering NICU team requested an ethics consultation at that point, and the on-call ethicist met with the patient's parents, whom he described in his note as "very loving." They felt that it would not be in their son's best interests to postpone what they believed to be his inevitable death by using burdensome treatments. This ethicist found their request for discontinuation of treatment to be "within a reasonable construal of parental discretion" and, thus, felt that it was ethically permissible to withdraw mechanical ventilation. The parents then sent the rest of the family home without informing them that support was to be withdrawn that evening, the patient died in his parents' arms soon after extubation.

The primary medical team, upon returning to work on Monday morning, expressed concern over the outcome. They felt excluded from the decision-making process and wondered whether the request for extubation had intentionally been made on a weekend because the parents had sensed the primary team's opposition to this course of action, particularly in light of the patient's recent improvement. An ethics consultant reviewed the case and ultimately concluded that he would have been unlikely to support withdrawal of mechanical ventilation at that time.

Professional reflections/lessons

Ethical dilemmas in pediatrics, particularly those involving limitation of life-sustaining treatment (LST), can be emotionally wrenching – neonatal cases, especially so. Pediatric patients referred for ethics consultation tend to be sicker than adult patients, and the question at hand more often deals with the limitation of life-sustaining treatment. Frequently, the consultant is called on to sanction, or even "bless," the family or medical team's decision to withdraw support.[1]

From an ethical point of view, in light of the fact that a newborn cannot (and never was able to) make autonomous decisions, medical decisions must be made according to the "best interests standard," as interpreted by the patient's parents or guardian. The question of what is in the patient's best interests – and the limits of parental latitude in determining this – has been pondered on. The topic became front page news in the 1970s as ethicists debated the matter and neonatologists acknowledged how many such newborns died as a result of withholding or withdrawing life-sustaining treatment.[2] In the 1980s, the Baby Doe rules famously restricted limitation of treatment to three specific situations: the patient is irreversibly comatose, the treatment itself is futile (in terms of survival), or is "virtually futile and inhumane."[3] The President's Commission for the Study of Ethical Problems in Medicine placed greater emphasis on the infant's projected quality of life and favored deferring to parental discretion, where the considered treatment was of uncertain benefit.[4]

Parental refusal of necessary treatments constitutes medical neglect, which health professionals are required to report to Child Protective Services (CPS). The threshold for reporting is not parental refusal of what the physician believes is the optimal course of treatment, however, on occasion, health professionals disagree with parents in this regard. Rather, reporting is justified where, in the physician's opinion, parental action is *clearly contrary to* the child's best interests.

The state generally intervenes only "where immediate action is necessary or where the potential for harm is rather serious."[5]

In the case being discussed, a CPS report was never a consideration mainly because the covering NICU team and on-call ethicist felt extubation was not contrary to the best interests of the patient. Such a report would only have fractured therapeutic relationships because it was no longer necessary to continue treatment. Had the covering team been aware of the concerns of the primary team, it could simply have deferred the decision until Monday morning when the latter returned.

Philosophers often say that "if you don't ask the right question, you'll never reach the right answer." In this case, there were two distinct yet related questions. The overarching question was how to balance parental rights and patient well-being (which the on-call ethicist chose to address); however, the urgent question of the weekend consult was whether to honor the parents' request for extubation on *that day*. Put simply, did immediate withdrawal of the ventilator fall within the bounds of parental discretion, either in terms of the Baby Doe rules (i.e., was continued treatment "virtually futile and inhumane") or the more permissive President's Commission recommendations concerning treatments of uncertain benefit? To this question, the hospital's two ethicists reached conflicting answers.

Haunting aspects

In clinical medicine, there exists a presumption (usually false) that there is one right course of action. Certainly, there are well-accepted algorithms, such as the resuscitation protocol for cardiac arrest, that define the appropriate response in a given situation. More often, however, clinical response permits a measure of latitude, such as in choosing between similar antibiotics.

Clinical ethicists ought not to harbor any delusions about the existence of one right course of action, for we are seldom involved in cases open to a single, clear answer. Ethics consultations are best reserved for ambiguous and value-laden situations where stakeholders disagree. These adjectives also describe clinical ethicists themselves, given the fervent disagreement within the field regarding both hot-button societal issues (e.g., embryonic stem-cell research) and specific patient-care dilemmas.[6] One would go so far as to *expect* an ethicist who prioritizes patient autonomy to disagree with one who emphasizes a beneficence-in-trust model of medical decision making. The "individual consultant model" of ethics consultation has, thus, been criticized for "[risking] unchecked ethical bias and the exclusion of other important participants in what should be a multidisciplinary process."[7] Although this model is considered highly efficient and nimble (in terms of response time to consult requests), this criticism is one of the reasons the model is used in only 9% of U.S. hospitals.[8]

It would be wise, then, for an institution that uses an individual consultant model to have an ethics committee available for exceedingly difficult cases. Such a forum exists in our institution, but a committee structure by its very nature is not conducive to urgent consultation for practical reasons of scheduling. An institution should also take steps to ensure a similar mindset among its ethicists, or at least a respect for institutional precedent, analogous to the legal concept of *stare decisis* ("to stand by that which is decided"). This would prevent ethicist A's recommendations from being consistently and substantively different than ethicist B's, thereby precluding a clinical team from, say, deferring consultations until the ethicist most likely to agree with them is on call.

What makes this case so troubling is that the two consultants in question do, in fact, agree on a vast array of issues. We are dear friends and faithful adherents of the same religious tradition. One (RDO) is the other's (RCM) mentor in clinical ethics, the secondary agent on his health-care proxy, even the "surrogate grandfather" to his children. It would not be going too far to say that RCM is a clinical ethicist because of RDO. In five years of working side-by-side, we have found that this case is one of only a handful of cases we have fundamentally disagreed on, and the one with the longest-reaching implications.

One reason for this professional disagreement is that only one of us actually took part in the consultation. Even a comprehensive written report or verbal recounting of events inevitably leaves out the unquantifiable and, perhaps, preconscious details that can sway a consultant in one direction. The parents in this case were described as "loving," but that word can mean so many different things, and a host of other adjectives could have been applied to them and the decision they faced. The colleague offering retrospective peer review can be more dispassionate and is protected from the risks taken by the active consultant, shielded from the grief in the parents' eyes and from the innocence of a newborn struggling for life.

It is certainly disturbing that the parents instructed the other relatives to leave without informing them that LST was about to be withdrawn, thus, casting doubt on the parents' motivations (or, at least, their confidence that they were doing the right thing). However, at the time of the consult, this had not yet happened and, if the on-call ethicist had been able to foresee that this would ensue, he likely would have shared these retrospective concerns. An ethicist who indulges in "if I knew then what I know now" ruminations will be driven to incapacitating self-doubt.

That the consultation was requested on Sunday afternoon is also significant, for quality-of-life reasons. Ethicists speak often about "quality of life," but they invariably apply the term to patients and families, never to themselves. Yet, just as the identity of the ethics consultant influences the outcome of the consultation, so does the timing. If the consult had not been called on a weekend, the on-call ethicist would have been more likely to run the case by his colleague. Moreover, if the consultation had been requested on a weekday, an impromptu convening of the ethics committee may have been possible. Much as we would like to deny it, all aspects of patient care suffer on weekends and holidays, as does ethics consultation.

The case haunts us to this day because it reflects the subjective – if not downright capricious – nature of ethics consultation. From peer-reviewed literature to casual conversation, the question is often raised as to what qualifies a person to be an "ethicist" and what right such a person has to proclaim what is ethical or not. Every ethicist has a practiced response to this indictment, often referencing his or her academic background and familiarity with ethical and legal principle. Ethicists may also point to their avowed facilitation approach (if applicable), whereby consensus is valued above fiat. Often, the inquisitor is not convinced; in reflecting on this case, neither are we.

Everything – given the inherent limitations of the "individual consultant" model – was done "right" in this case. The on-call ethicist is experienced and thoughtful, a person committed to upholding the integrity of ethics consultation. The family and medical staff were interviewed, and relevant legal and ethical precedents were considered. Consensus among all present was even achieved. Yet, is it possible that everyone agreed on the wrong answer? For if the consultation had been requested on a different day, the conclusions could have been different. The patient may even be alive today. If our ethical recommendations fluctuate so significantly, based on personality or day of the week, perhaps we clinical ethicists really do not qualify as members of a "discipline" after all.

If we confess to epistemic limitations in one respect, we must be consistent throughout. For even if the patient were still alive on that Monday, he might not be today. Perhaps, months of burdensome treatment would have ensued until it was finally clear even to the reviewing ethicist as it long had been to the parents – that the child was suffering unnecessarily. Or, perhaps, placed in that situation, and staring into the vacant eyes of a mother and father making the hardest decision anyone could make, that ethicist would have authorized withdrawal, too. Then, the roles would have been reversed, and the reviewing ethicist would have been the one questioned in an *ex post facto* conference (not to mention a book chapter) by a friend and colleague; each of us would still be haunted by this case, but for opposite reasons.

Not infrequently, hospital staff – some of whom we do not know particularly well, and many with stressful roles, on whom lives frequently depend – will stop us in the hallway and say, for no apparent reason, "I'm sure glad I don't have your job." Our responses often vary: sometimes a sardonic laugh; occasionally, a witty retort. In the days following this consultation, we usually just nodded in agreement.

Outcome

A few weeks after the patient's death, a meeting was held that included both ethics consultants, the covering and primary neonatologists, the NICU social worker, and a representative from CPS. Although some felt that an appropriate decision had been made, others felt that further review – whether a full ethics committee meeting or notification of CPS – would have allowed divergent opinions to be heard and the baby's prognosis to potentially become clearer. Some suggested that pursuing an ethics consultation earlier would have been beneficial, not only for the NICU team but also for the parents and even the ethicist himself (whoever that happened to be on the given day). The on-call ethicist expressed the sentiment that he wished he had taken the time to consult a colleague prior to offering recommendations.

Several systems-level "next steps" were identified. The neonatologists stated their intention to encourage the NICU nursing staff to include clinical ethics in their regular in-services and to involve the Department of Clinical Ethics more routinely (and earlier on) in complex cases such as this one. Both ethicists affirmed their willingness to participate in challenging cases even when not on call and expressed the hope that fuller committee involvement would be possible in such situations.

On a more personal level, three lessons learned should be mentioned. First, for all the politically correct embracing of the facilitation approach to ethics consultation, in the end, consensus is not always reliable. Sometimes the ethics consultant has to follow the lead of Henry Fonda in 12 *Angry Men* and be the lone holdout against (what he believes to be) the wrong course of action. This may involve looking disconsolate parents in the eye and telling them you cannot honor their request, no matter how deeply you empathize with their pain (the very reason so many are glad they do not have this job). Yet, all the while you hold on to a sliver of hope that a right consensus will be reached – through benefit of time, discussion, and reflection – just like in the movies.[9]

Second, at the conclusion of every ethics consultation, one should "come up for air." It is easy to get so immersed in the medical details, ethical arguments, and legal precedents of a case that one forgets to consider something obvious and critical. Before completing a write-up or rendering an opinion, the consultant should take a deep breath and check to make sure that he has not overlooked something. In this case, that something could have been distinguishing between the larger question and the pressing question, thereby putting the option of deferring a decision until the primary NICU team returned back on the table. For the most difficult cases, the final review should be done in tandem, with the benefit of a colleague's feedback and perspective.

Finally, clinical ethics, like any other discipline, is a profoundly human endeavor. With the benefit of hindsight, many expressed regret that life support was withdrawn from this child, at least without the input of the physicians and nurses who knew him best. And although it is tempting to blame such an outcome on an ethics consultation deficient in preparation, process, or experience, such was not the case here. Even the most competent ethicist will eventually tender a recommendation that, in retrospect, he will come to question and, perhaps, even regret. The degree to which he learns from such an experience, and has the courage to enter the ethical fray once more, has more to do with character and dedication than with education and qualifications.

Discussion questions

1. At your institution, do patients receive optimal care (including ethics consultation) at all times, including nights, weekends, holidays? If not, how can we better balance professionals' own "quality of life" with that of patients?
2. Are there "right answers" to clinical ethical questions? (Or, are there always wrong answers?) If so, why do ethicists so often disagree? If not, does clinical ethics deserve to be considered a "discipline"?
3. How important is precedent in the work of an ethics consultation service? In other words, if a previous consultation recommended a certain course of action, can a consultant offer a different recommendation in a similar case?
4. When colleagues fundamentally disagree on a case, what is the best forum for discussion so that neither feels judged nor accused? In what way can we improve practice through peer review?

REFERENCES

1. Orr RD, Perkin RM. Clinical ethics consultations with children. *J Clin Ethics*, 1994; 5(4): 323–8.
2. Duff RS, Campbell AG. Moral and ethical dilemmas in the special care nursery. *New Engl J Med*, 1973; 289(17): 890–4.
3. Nondiscrimination on the basis of handicap; procedures and guidelines relating to health care for handicapped infants – HHS. Final rules. *Fed Regist*, 1985; 50: 14879–92.
4. President's Commission for the Study of Ethical Problems in Medicine and Biomedical and Behavioral Research. *Deciding to forgo life-sustaining treatment.* Washington, DC: U.S. Government Printing Office, 1983.
5. Wing KR. The law and the public's health, 3rd ed. Ann Arbor, MI: Health Administration Press, 1990; 32. (As quoted in Diekema DS. Parental refusals of medical treatment: the harm principle as threshold for state intervention. *Theor Med*, 2004; 25(4): 250–1.)
6. Fox E, Stocking C. Ethics consultants' recommendations for life-prolonging treatment of patients in a persistent vegetative state. *JAMA*, 1993; 270(21): 2578–82.
7. Fletcher JC, Hoffman DE. Ethics committees: time to experiment with standards. *Ann Intern Med*, 1994; 120(4): 335–8.
8. Fox E, Meyers S, Pearlman R. Ethics consultation in U.S. hospitals: a national survey. *AJOB*, 2007; 7(2): 13–25.
9. *12 Angry Men*. MGM Studios, 1957.

2

When a baby dies in pain

Thomas R. McCormick and David Woodrum

Case narrative

Baby Zelda was delivered by C-section at 25 weeks of gestation to an 18-year-old first-time mother. The pregnancy was complicated by a maternal urinary tract infection, prolonged ruptured amniotic membranes, amnionitis, and fetal distress. The infant required aggressive resuscitation that included oxygen, tracheal intubation, and assisted ventilation. Following successful resuscitation and stabilization, the infant was admitted to the neonatal intensive care unit (NICU). Support measures included oxygen, assisted ventilation, parenteral maintenance of fluids and nutrition, antibiotics, red blood cell transfusions, and analgesia. Unfortunately, Baby Zelda's respiratory status deteriorated, requiring increased oxygen and ventilator support. She was also hypotensive, so pressors were added. Toward the end of the first week of life, she developed signs of necrotizing entercolitis (NEC), a potentially serious complication of prematurity involving the immature gastrointestinal tract.[1] Zelda's necrotizing entercolitis progressed and her condition reached the point that surgical intervention, with a view toward resection of the damaged bowel, was necessary. However, at surgery the extent of bowel involvement appeared to be too great to permit definitive resection. Accordingly, as is the standard of care in such cases, the abdomen was closed. Aggressive medical care was continued and a "second look" was planned in several days. The second look showed that most of the patient's bowel was irreversibly damaged. Any attempt to remove the involved area would leave Zelda with a much shortened, nonfunctional bowel – incompatible with long-term survival.

In a postsurgery conference, the surgeons and NICU team counseled the family, relaying that there was no definitive treatment for the baby's condition, no chance for survival, and a 100% risk of suffering. Zelda's caretakers, particularly the bedside nurses, estimated that the infant's quality of life was extremely poor and her degree of suffering was great, "as bad as anyone can remember for a patient in this NICU." Moreover, aggressive and escalating pain management was not working. Zelda continued to experience great pain. The entire care team believed that the goal of therapy should change from curative to palliative care. They recommended withdrawing aggressive life support and initiating all palliative measures so Baby Zelda could live out her short life as comfortably as possible.

Zelda's parents responded to the conference by verbalizing disbelief and doubt about the team's prognosis and insisted that aggressive care continue. Zelda's mother exclaimed, "You all are wrong, my baby is going to live! I haven't had anything in my life except this baby, and you are not taking her away from me!" After several days of discussion and disagreement between the care team and the infant's parents, we were called for an ethics consultation.

Professional reflections

We discussed this case with all of the parties involved over a period of several days. As healthcare professionals with a strong motivation to help others, it is only natural to feel a sense of compassion for the suffering of these parents as well as for the suffering of this premature baby. Likewise, we empathized with the immediate caregivers' suffering as they attended to a baby they could not heal but could only attend to through a protracted and painful process of dying.

When healthcare providers see the wisdom of a transition from aggressive intervention to palliative and comfort care of a child, it requires a major shift in the goals and expectations of the parents. Most parents feel a sense of responsibility to advocate for the survival of their child. Thus, disagreements often arise, and the situation becomes problematic for the healthcare provider who is taught to ensure that decisions are made in the "best interest" of the infant patient, or, as Diekema suggests, ensuring that decisions minimize harm to the patient.[2,3] Specifically, Baby Zelda suffered from the discomfort of the usual intensive care interventions and from progressive bowel necrosis and peritonitis.

Even though as ethics consultants we were called upon to render our services with relative objectivity, we could not avoid the conclusion that this tiny patient was experiencing great suffering due to her underlying condition with no anticipation of pleasurable experiences and no hope for survival. Empathically, we felt drawn into the suffering of not only the patient but also the parents. Nevertheless, our task was to maintain our professional objectivity and to focus our attention primarily on the "best interests" of this vulnerable and dependent patient.

From our perspective, Baby Zelda's suffering was disproportionate to any benefit obtained by the continuation of life support. In such cases, healthcare professionals are guided by the principle of proportionality, requiring that burdens of treatment be justified by the benefits accruing to the patient. When the burdens far outweigh the benefits, the goals of medicine most often shift from curative to palliative. Consideration should also be given to the "do no harm" principle. Beauchamp and Childress comment on Gerald Kelly's explanation of proportionality: "For a therapy to be obligatory or required, it must (a) offer a *reasonable prospect* of benefit, and (b) not involve *excessive* expense, pain, or other inconvenience. The substance of the distinction is a balance between benefit and detriment."[4]

After considerable discussion with all parties, we concurred with the team that the most appropriate ethical approach in this particular case would be a shift to palliative care. When a longtime neonatologist (DW) is serving in the role of a consultant on an NICU case, it is not hard to imagine oneself as the attending physician in the case. Still, the very nature of the situation requires that the consultants maintain the "moral point of view," and by that we mean remaining dispassionate, as objective as possible, respecting the perspectives of all the stake-holders while seeking an ethical resolution to the major conflict in the case that is congruent with our guiding ethical principles. The second consultant (TMC), a bioethicist with a long history of teaching residents and consulting in the NICU, provided a second pair of eyes and ears in examining the perspectives of all involved and thus opened a second point of dialogue in sorting through the issues and moving to a recommendation. Both consultants agreed with the unanimous recommendation of the treating team. Despite the ethics consultants' support for the ethical soundness of a shift to palliative care, the parents persisted in their insistence that everything be done to prolong and save the life of their baby.

The nursing staff was devastated by the parents' decision. Some nurses requested that they not be assigned to Baby Zelda as the infant's suffering was too upsetting for them. It seemed to us that the primary nurses who were caring for the baby were experiencing what is often referred to as "moral distress," that is, being a participant in a morally tragic situation yet lacking the power to change the situation. These nurses felt a strong duty to protect Baby Zelda. The American Nurses Association (ANA) Code (2001) emphasizes the importance of this professional duty: "The nurse promotes, advocates for, and strives to protect the health, safety and rights of the patient." These nurses believed there was a conflict between their professional duties as defined in the ANA Code of Ethics and the duties they were called upon to perform by the demands of the parents.[5] Both consultants could understand and sympathize with the predicament of these nurses. After all, the nurses are the ones at the bedside of such babies 24 hours of each day.

We empathized as well with the medical staff. Each time members of the staff rounded they again faced the baby's predicament as well as the nurses' distress. The attending in this case wondered aloud whether to seek a court opinion allowing the hospital to discontinue the use of the ventilator on the grounds that it was "futile" to continue using it. He raised an interesting question, which was considered numerous times as the treating team watched Zelda's "futile" suffering.

Although the NICU staff wondered about the futility of life support in this case, there is a consensus that invoking the concept of futility in pediatrics today is essentially a nonissue. Lantos claims: "As a practical and legal matter, the controversy has been essentially resolved. There are virtually no situations in which courts will give permission to doctors to withhold or withdraw treatment that parents request.

Instead, courts have allowed parents to demand intubation of anencephalic babies and continued home ventilation of brain-dead children."[6]

In the authors' view palliative care and a natural death are what "ought to have been done." Yet there remains the procedural question of who should control that decision. The court has a considerable number of precedent cases on which it could base a decision regarding a court mandate for intervention intended to save the patient's life. (Transfusions of minors against parental wishes were tested in *Jehovah's Witnesses vs. King County [Harborview]*).[7] The law is fairly clear: Lifesaving transfusions can be given to minors against parental wishes![8]

On the other hand, in the case of Baby Zelda, precedent might be expected to influence a court decision that would deny overriding the parents' wishes – not addressing what "should be done" but rather "who should decide." If the court addresses only the later procedural question it may simply conclude that in such controversies the parents have the right to decide because they are categorically defined as decision-makers for their minor children.[7]

Additionally, although from different legal perspectives (basing their judgment on the *Emergency Treatment and Active Labor Act 42 U.S.C. Sec. 1395dd* and the Baby Doe regulations), in the instances of Baby K (an anencephalic infant) and Baby Ryan (a former premature infant with conditions thought by the medical community to be incompatible with survival) the courts mandated continued aggressive life-supportive care.[9,10]

Ethics consultations often focus on disagreements between providers and surrogate decision-makers. The background and the reasons for such disagreements can stem from several factors: (a) There have been dramatic improvements in survival and outcome from all sorts of formerly lethal neonatal conditions, such as extreme prematurity or major congenital defects, and these have been well documented in the lay press. These reports, along with television vignettes that tend to feature so-called "miracle babies," often lead to unrealistic expectations from parents when they read about these well-publicized "miracles." (b) The emergence of personal autonomy in medical decision making has altered the parent/physician relationship. Now, when it comes to end-of-life situations, parents may feel authorized to demand that their wishes be carried out against medical advice. For example, in spite of good-faith efforts to point out facial grimaces and writhing movements of Zelda's body that we believed to be in response to her painful condition, the parents were either unable to recognize or did not interpret these signs as indications of pain and suffering. Therefore, there was an ongoing difference of perception about the suffering of the baby between the parents and the professional staff that continued throughout this infant's brief lifetime. (c) Parents and providers proceed from different perspectives; for example, the healthcare team may be responding primarily to medical and prognostic factors while the parents may be relying on personal values, spiritual or cultural beliefs, and their desperate hope for survival. (d) Finally, by the time an ethics consult is called for, often trust between family and staff has broken down. One of the benefits of an ethics consultation is that all parties feel they have a new and neutral party to communicate with, and a richer, fuller description of the case and its complexities can usually be obtained. Often, the process of carrying out a consultation contributes to a consensual resolution because it enables a higher level of communication and contributes to a higher level of mutual understanding. As consultants, we entered the case with an expectation that by listening carefully to the thoughts and feelings of all parties, by obtaining the relevant facts of the case, and by recognizing the values and goals of the various stakeholders we could contribute to a good resolution of the conflicts. However, this was not to be the case. The extreme degree of suffering by Zelda, her hopeless survival potential, and the refusal of her parents to perceive or acknowledge either were unique.

Haunting aspects

The case of Baby Zelda haunts us because of the profound suffering of everyone involved. The NICU social worker, despite a long and successful career as a patient advocate, was rejected by Zelda's parents and felt that she failed them. The physicians involved, despite great efforts, could "help" neither Zelda nor her parents negotiate the inevitable dying process. The NICU nurses were profoundly affected by their inability to alleviate Zelda's suffering and by the hostile attitude of her parents toward them.

Clearly, Zelda's parents suffered. They were self-described as poor and used to living a simple rural life. Their exposure to the medical system was limited, and their reaction to the high-tech urban referral center was guardedly suspicious. Moreover, after counseling by the NICU team, the attitudes of this couple might be more accurately characterized as mistrustful and hostile. Indeed, they began visiting only in the middle of the night to avoid the NICU staff.

Perhaps the most haunting issue of concern for the authors was the sustained suffering of Baby Zelda. As the bowel necrosis and attendant peritonitis progressed, Zelda's abdominal distension increased. Fluid and gas accumulated, and the suture line from the previous surgical incisions threatened to split. Aggressive use of analgesic agents was considered by the bedside providers to be insufficient.

Outcome

The conclusion of the ethics consultation process that took place over several days was more supportive of the NICU staff position (i.e., Baby Zelda should receive palliative, end-of-life comfort care) than of the parents, who demanded continued aggressive life-support care. Because of the strong feelings surrounding this case, the consultants brought the case to a meeting of the full ethics committee, which concurred with the initial recommendation of the consultant team. The ethics committee's rationale was essentially the same as the consultants': (a) consensus prognosis for survival was nil and (b) there was clear evidence of severe ongoing suffering by the infant. Clearly, in the eyes of all involved, except the parents, the benefit of further life support was minimal and the burden on the baby was excessive.

It was no surprise to anyone that the parents of Baby Zelda did not concur with the ethics committee's recommendation. In our experience, the consultation process usually results in a consensus agreement between the involved parties. After several days of further stalemate the matter was referred to the hospital administrators for consideration as to whether the *parens patriae* approach to the infant's best interest/no harm should be implemented. (The state has a latent parental role concerning its vulnerable citizens that might be invoked for the protection of the baby.[2]) The hospital administration surveyed case law throughout the country and concluded that a referral to the court was in all likelihood doomed to failure. Accordingly, supportive care was continued in compliance with the parents' request and with renewed emphasis on pain control. The infant lived for several more days before dying on life-support systems.

In hindsight, we now believe it was not appropriate for members of the medical staff to consider going to court to resolve this particular case as it may have kindled a false hope that a court-based solution could be found and would have fostered a somewhat adversarial relationship. In any similar future cases, if staff mentions the possibility of going to court, we will actively discourage this notion and share our rationale as described above. The energy of the staff is best used in communicating with the parents of the infant, developing a relationship with them, and deepening our understanding of their thoughts, feelings, and values. A deepening trust might have led the parents to a clearer insight into the nature of their infant's suffering; however, we remain perplexed as to how we might have accomplished that goal. Even if the parents did not come to such a conclusion, it is important that the staff not abandon them but give them the benefit of the doubt that they are most likely doing the best they can under these stressful circumstances. This case highlights a situation where the parents subjectively feel they are making the right choice while others believe there is objective evidence to the contrary. Such cases challenge us as consultants to maintain our empathy with the parents while working to ensure the best interests of the infant.

Discussion questions

1. What should the ethics consultant do when the parents do not agree with a care plan designed in the baby's best interest and will not consent for the plan considered optimal by the attending physician? Is it ever advantageous (morally acceptable) to involve the courts in these kinds of decisions?

2. Should ethics consultants routinely bring cases of this nature to the ethics committee? Why or why not?
3. When is it the role of the ethics consultant to be "objective"? Does personal emotion enrich or denigrate ethical decision making in cases?
4. How should we weigh the stakeholders' perception of the infant's suffering against the parents' view? Should the parents' view ever trump the healthcare professional's? What is the ethics consultant's role in determining who has such final authority?

REFERENCES

1. Taeusch HW, Ballard RA, eds. *Avery's Diseases of the Newborn*, 8th ed. Philadelphia: Elsevier-Saunders, 2005; 1123–32.
2. President's Commission for the Study of Ethical Problems in Medicine and Biomedical and Behavioral Research. *Deciding to Forgo Life-Sustaining Treatment.* Washington, DC: U.S. Government Printing Office, 1983.
3. Diekema DS. Parental refusal of medical treatment: The harm principle and threshold for state intervention. *Theor Med,* 2004; 25: 243–64.
4. Beauchamp T, Childress J. *Principles of Biomedical Ethics*, 5th ed. Oxford: Oxford University Press, 2001; 124.
5. Schroeter K. Ethics in perioperative practice – patient advocacy. *AORN J,* 2002; 75(5): 941–4, 949.
6. Lantos J. When parents request seemingly futile treatment for their children. *Mt Sinai J Med,* 2006; 73(3): 587.
7. *The Revised Code of Washington* 7.70.065.
8. Groudine SB. The child Jehovah's Witness patient: A legal and ethical dilemma. *Surgery,* 1997; 121: 357–8.
9. Capron AM. At law: Baby Ryan and virtual futility. *The Hastings Cent Rep,* 1995; 25: 2.
10. Annas GJ. Asking the courts to set the standard of emergency care – the case of Baby K. *New Engl J Med,* 2006; 330: 1542–5.

3

But how *can* we choose?

Richard M. Zaner

Case narrative

I had been at the medical center only a short time when I was asked by one of the physicians in the maternal–fetal unit to consult on what was said to be an "abortion" problem. A 22-year-old married woman, I was told, a Mrs. Judy Nelson, had been referred by her own obstetrician for evaluation and management of her first pregnancy, which was thought to be problematic, although the obstetrician was unsure precisely how to read the several ultrasounds (US) she had performed. Mrs. Nelson's pregnancy was thought to be about 22 ± 2 weeks gestational age.

Physicians and specialists in our maternal–fetal unit confirmed the estimated fetal age. They also noted a myelomeningocele, however, along with possible ventricular dilatation – "spina bifida" with patent spinal lesion and protrusion. Presumably, Mrs. Nelson's own obstetrician had seen enough to refer her to our unit, although uncertainty made her reluctant to tell her patient very much.

Informed of these results, the woman was also told that the radiologists could not be "completely certain" of many aspects of that diagnosis; for greater accuracy, serial USs – several taken over a week or so – would be needed to determine whether, beyond the spinal protrusion, the apparent hydrocephalus was growing worse.

The woman was told she faced several options in light of the diagnosis by the maternal–fetal specialist who had taken her case. On the one hand, she could "continue with the pregnancy," but if developing hydrocephalus were to become clear, there was a "real chance" that she would have to undergo a cesarian. When she asked why that might happen, she was told that the fetal head size might preclude vaginal delivery.

Clearly stunned by this news, she was immediately informed that there was another option: abortion, described as a "therapeutic option."

"What do you mean, 'abortion?'" she demanded.

A version of this chapter was originally published in *The Journal of Clinical Ethics*, 16 (3): 218–22. ©2005 by *The Journal of Clinical Ethics*. Used with permission. All rights reserved.

A bit taken aback by her tone and demeanor, the physician, who relayed this to me later, pointed out, "Well, you see, it's what is described as . . ."

"'Described as?' What in the world does *that* mean?"

"Well, you see, if you'll just give me a chance to say it . . ." As he said to me, he was at the same time confused by her insistent questions and beginning to get a bit nervous over what she was really trying to say to him. It seemed pretty evident to him, he told me, that she was already quite upset, and she seemed to be getting ever more angry.

"So, say it, then: What is this all about? I mean, there I was, all happy and warm and my baby on the way, and then I'm told to just come here and see what's going on, and I don't know what that's all about . . ."

"What it's all about is that our ultrasound techs have seen what they believe is spina bifida, and I understand that they talked with you about what that is, what it means, and so on."

"Sure, they talked about that, and they mentioned that other thing, that hydro thing . . ."

"Hydrocephalus."

"Right, that, and well, then you come along and talk about 'described as' and 'there's a chance,' and then talk about abortion . . ."

As the physician continued, more carefully, more gently, to tell her why there may be a need to abort, and that the gestational age of her fetus was rapidly approaching the "cutoff" date, she only grew more and more agitated. When he pointed out that "state law prohibits abortions after 24 weeks gestation" – without, he added, a documented threat to her own life – she just "exploded."

"What exactly made you think she was 'exploding,'" I asked when we first discussed the consult.

"I don't know what else you'd call it," he explained. "I mean, she grew red in the face, her voice escalated way up the scale, and she, well, she just exploded – no other word for it."

She was rapidly approaching that cutoff date; in fact, if serial ultrasounds were performed, she might well go beyond the date before "developing hydrocephalus" could be confirmed or disconfirmed. It was at this point that he had backed off, sensing what he took to be "real anger" at him, and told her that he would get "someone" to talk with her. So, there she sat, by herself in the so-called "quiet room," waiting for "someone" to explain everything and, it was hoped, to help calm her down.

"I also pointed out," he said, "that an alpha-fetoprotein (AFP) test might be helpful, with results known within a day or so – still well within the time left before the cutoff date."

"Was it done?"

"Well, sure, of course, we had to do it, you know?"

"So, OK, then, but what results?"

"Don't know yet, but they should be back today sometime."

The test had been done, and she was at this moment awaiting both him and the results. So, I had to be sure not to get ahead of the tests but still begin addressing what needed attention.

When I got to her room, someone, a nurse as I recall, was already there and they were talking about the AFP test results. I waited in the hall for a few moments until the nurse came out. She saw me and told me that she had informed the woman that the AFP was positive for a neural-tube defect. She made a point of telling the woman that results from these tests were not 100% certain. Indeed, she had emphasized that test results show a "statistically significant" number of false positives (as well as false negatives).

"You know, she is really upset, Mrs. Nelson."

"What do you mean?"

"I mean she is upset; I'm not even sure she understood what I told her."

I stepped into her room, noted her husband was also there, and introduced myself to them. I was met with both glares and tears. Clearly agitated, they nevertheless seemed quite willing to talk with me.

"Anything," she said straight off, "anything that can help clear up this mess."

"Mess?"

"I don't know what else you'd call it," she said. "I mean, what is this, can't anybody be straight about this? I thought that coming here and seeing all these specialists, so-called, I'd get some answers. But all I get is 'maybe this' and 'maybe that,' and 'perhaps,' and, my lord, nothing straight, all these dodges, all this 'we're not sure' and . . ."

"Whoa," I broke in. "Maybe, Mr. and Mrs. Nelson, we'd better try and see what's been going on, what you've been told, why you're so angry."

Talking with the couple, she was obviously agitated, anxious, and angry, as was he, though not as much. But not at the doctor. I told them that my role was to help them think carefully about their situation in light of their own beliefs and, for that, I had to listen to what they had to say.

They obviously understood matters quite well. They knew, for instance, that if the pregnancy continued, and hydrocephalus was severe, there was a good chance that labor might have to be induced before full term, probably by cesarean (because of fetal head size), with neonatal care thereafter: shunting the hydrocephalus, surgery to close the spinal lesion, ventilator assistance, etc.

Rarely do you find such clarity or intelligence, I thought to myself. Still, there was something else bothering them. She asked: "Put yourself in our shoes: We know we've got to decide, but it's just not fair to ask this when things are not clear!"

Haunting aspects

The problem was clearly not abortion, neither for them nor for the physician. As evident as it was compelling, the issue posed a harsh dilemma for them. Any decision they could make would be irreversible (even not deciding would soon be set in stone, with the 24-week date coming up soon), yet it could only be based on information at once uncertain and confusing.

"How," Mr. Nelson blurted out, "can anybody be asked to make such a decision when the tests could be wrong?"

His wife asked, "But how can we decide to continue with the pregnancy if the tests are right? I know they're only trying to do their best," she continued plaintively, "But the way they talk, we don't know what to think. Once we've decided, we can't 'undecide,' and the basis for it is just not certain enough for that kind of decision. For that, you ought to be able to be more certain!"

My observation, given as gently and sincerely as it could be, went something like this: "Isn't moral life like that? Most often very critical matters have to be decided when we're not entirely sure either of the basis or the consequences." My opening remark was received with understanding and anguish. They also probed the options if the pregnancy were continued and the baby did have patent spina bifida, as well as the other possibilities if it did not or if the spinal lesions were minor (an almost normal baby). The important thing was for them to be very clear that they really had thought about each of the possibilities as thoroughly as they could at this time, so that in the aftermath no matter what decision they made they would be less likely to berate themselves with thoughts of "if only we had . . ." – that is, experience subsequent guilt, anger, and resentment.

"You mean," Mrs. Nelson responded, "that all we can do is just decide, even if it turns out we are wrong?"

"No, perhaps it means that you have to try and figure out just what they're telling you about the US and the AFP test. They said there is a 'statistically significant chance' that the AFP was a 'false positive,' and that the radiologists were '75% confident' of their interpretation."

"But what does all that mean?" Mr. Nelson asked.

"Well," I responded, "if 'statistically significant' is translated, it means something like, oh, maybe 3–5%."

"What?" she broke in. "Doesn't that mean that there is a 95% to 97% chance the test is *right*?"

"Not only that," I responded. "The radiologists think their reading is very likely correct – 3 out of 4 chances. Put that together with the AFP test. Both are more likely correct than not."

Mrs. Nelson at one point exclaimed: "The doctor just doesn't understand what it's like for us." In almost the same breath, she seemed to plead: "Put yourself in our shoes: Is it right to force a baby to be a hero just to stay alive . . .?" This was also meant for the doctor to understand "what it's like for us."

Not to belabor the obvious, she was urgently asking the doctor at once *to understand* and, more importantly, *to be understanding*. The sense in which they conveyed this was powerful and heart-rending. How difficult it was for them to face the irreversibility of what they knew was necessary yet could hardly, if ever, be justified. Is an ethics that truly takes account of uncertainty possible? Can it be anything else?

For that matter, and more personally, I was left with a strong sense of my own vulnerability in the face of such uncertainty. I know I have often used the words, thinking I knew what they really meant: We have got to have an ethics that is responsive to the realities of genuine uncertainty, vagueness, not knowing what seems necessary in order to decide, much less to act. But do I understand? I know that the Nelsons brought home a sense that, in truth, I probably did not understand, even while I know that they were grateful for this chance to talk, to open up, to share their own vulnerability. And so I am left with this – what shall I call it? This sense of my own not knowing just what is best for them or for me.

Professional reflections

This situation involved a relationship among different persons, each with their own experiences and interpretations. The sense of that relationship became apparent contextually. Although textured by their different feelings and thoughts, each of the individuals felt caught up in a kind of perilous adventure. Their respective involvements had the sense of uncertain and forbidding paths and eventualities, of a troubling trial or test. To listen to the wife's words, for instance, was to be immediately alerted to hazards faced by her baby and by them and to be alerted to their sense of not knowing what to do. Implicit in the equally passionate words of the doctor about their anger was also an alert – "watch out when you're dealing with this couple, for they are given to anger" – and a clear warning that since abortion was the presumed "problem," one needed to be on guard for the well-known controversies abortion always provokes.

Their various conversational and physiognomic expressions were thus marked at the outset with harbingers of possible pitfalls and precarious risks. But there was more to it. Their poignant plea for help in understanding things and reaching a decision, for instance, made their sense of vulnerability prominent. Though *they* had to make the decision, they had to trust *others* – the doctor and the radiologists – for vital information without which no right, good, or just decision could be made. The doctor, on the other hand, was cautious yet impatient – which may account for their sense that he was trying to "push" them to abortion. Yet he was confident that the diagnosis was correct, and he was in fact somewhat disturbed that things were not immediately obvious to the couple.

That peculiar mixture of caution and impatience was doubtless communicated to the couple. It certainly became a permanent part of my own understanding of the complications implicit in clinical life. It may also have been responsible for their reactions, which were seen by the doctor as "anger" toward him, as well as for their sense that "the doctor just doesn't understand what it's like for us."

This relationship thus turns out to be fundamental to apprehending the moral dimension of such encounters.

The issue of every consultation, I am led to conclude, is extraordinary caution, for what illness always bodes – more in its serious forms, of course – is the shattering of the ill person's world. It is also an appeal to others, the consultant in particular, to help remoralize and normalize what has been shattered. This means listening to those who are sick as they talk their way through their circumstances, thus recognizing the need to help "create conditions for [stories] to occur."[1]

Like many clinical encounters, this situation was remarkable for the range of passionate feelings (wishes, aims, hopes, etc.) variously expressed by the main characters. These feelings reveal remarkable significance. In the first place, the feelings manifested were evoked strictly by the fetus' condition (to a lesser degree, the parents'), were directed to the fetus as "now presented," and were aimed at the range of possible future prospects (as efforts to "do something" for the fetus and parents). In this complex sense, the feelings were *oriented* expressions of moral concern: efforts to do the right thing, to be good people, and to act fairly regarding everyone concerned. They were efforts to be responsive to the present (the now-presented and diagnosed fetus) and responsible for the future (the fetus and themselves as parents, whether the aftermath were abortion or an impaired infant).

Of course, something inevitably falls out of this for any clinical ethics consultation. What Arthur Frank says about illness narratives, or what he terms "telling-illness," is also true for those of us who tell stories about illnesses suffered by others. To undergo illness is to undergo an uprooting of the natural attitude – that quiet, unquestioning acceptance of "things as they are," which Alfred Schutz insisted is fundamental to social life.[2] In Frank's compelling words:

The loss of the taken-for-granted world – being wrenched out of the natural attitude and facing the fundamental anxiety of death – induces panic, in the mythic sense of unexpectedly encountering the terrifying god who screams in despair.[3]

Outcome

It was hardly surprising that the couple eventually settled on terminating the pregnancy. I say "settled on" because they were hardly content with this decision; it was not what they wanted, it was, as she said at one point, "what has to be done." The Nelsons had a strong conviction that it was "just not right," as Mrs. Nelson explained, that any baby should be forced to live with the severe defects their baby would have to face if it made it all the way to birth.

So they agreed to abort the pregnancy. They were deeply saddened by this but felt that there were just no other options. No one who had been involved with them were in any way happy with the outcome. But as the attending physician had emphasized, they could still plan on another pregnancy. True enough, I suppose, and quite possibly a good thing for them. I do not know if they ever actually did get pregnant again. I assume they did. Like so many clinical encounters, we were all left with a lot we did not and could not know. This is the pathos, I once said to myself, of clinical work.

Discussion questions

1. How can the ethics consultant correct for any serious misunderstandings? To what extent is it the consultant's role to do so?
2. Complex feelings and values require interpretation. How do consultants best "truthfully" relay these values to clinicians?
3. What constitutes "respect" in such complex consultations? How does/should the consultant convey respect to the couple? To the physician?

REFERENCES

1. The first published account of this story appeared in *J Clin Ethics*, Fall 2005; pp. 218–22.
2. Schutz A. Symbol, reality and society. In: Natanson M, ed. *Alfred Schutz: Collected Papers I.* The Hague: Martinus Nijhoff, 1971; 287–356.
3. Frank A. Experiencing illness through storytelling. In: Toombs SK, ed. *Handbook of Phenomenology and Medicine.* Dordrecht and Boston: Kluwer, 2001; 241.

4

Maternal–fetal surgery and the "profoundest question in ethics"

Mark J. Bliton

Narrative

I am thinking about Rebecca, her mother, and her fetus. For several years now, I have periodically found myself remembering our last encounter. Perhaps it is more accurate to say that I revisit certain images, seeking to understand a signature moral problem.

Rebecca had traveled to our hospital seeking information about maternal–fetal surgery to repair fetal spina bifida. One of the most morally intriguing surgeries in medicine over the past decade, it has stimulated considerable controversy as well as the need to examine the complicated, contested, and serious ethical issues it raises.[1,2,3] Some have argued, for example, that maternal–fetal surgery to repair fetal myelomeningocele should never be offered because it presents no medical benefit to the woman and not enough for the fetus.[3] There is some truth to this position because there is a 12% risk of premature delivery under 30-weeks' gestation, including a 5% risk of fetal or neonatal demise.[4] On the other hand, there has been sufficient indication of benefit to warrant a multi-center randomized clinical study funded by the National Institute of Child Health and Human Development to evaluate and possibly answer questions about the surgery's benefits. That study is currently open and ongoing.[5]

I meet with all women considering maternal–fetal surgery at my institution to address the many ethical issues and controversies. In these meetings, I try to help family members anticipate, identify, and understand the many personal, medical, social, and ethical issues they will face whether or not they decide to have the fetal repair.[6,7] Rebecca and her mother arrived when fetal repair was offered as an elective option. Accordingly, several identifiable moral factors deserve mention in Rebecca's case.

Having found out at approximately 18 weeks gestation that her fetus had spina bifida, Rebecca had already faced a choice about whether to continue or to terminate her pregnancy; she chose the former. In effect, she had made a decision to treat the spinal lesion, either by the standard way right after birth or by choosing open-uterine surgical repair. Her mother, who was supportive, accompanied Rebecca to her meetings with me (as well as to other meetings) because Rebecca's boyfriend had left when she decided to continue the pregnancy. I discussed the maternal and fetal risks associated with this open-uterine surgery, first with Rebecca, then with Rebecca and her mother, and then with both during a summary consultation with key members of the maternal–fetal surgery team.

Rebecca's vulnerability stood out in each of those meetings. Like many people, she had very little, if any, prior knowledge of or experience with spina bifida. Of course, she put her best face forward. Nevertheless, similar to many of the women with whom I have met, Rebecca demonstrated shock, confusion, a sense of loss, and anxiety about the choices she needed to make. There was much to consider about the anticipated future of her child-to-be. Little certainty could be offered beyond the likelihood of catheters, ankle or leg braces, a shunt for hydro-cephalus, other surgical procedures, numerous hospitalizations, and eventually a wheelchair.[8] I remember talking about her expectations of fetal repair – beneficial results were uncertain – even as she tearfully described her fears about the cognitive deficits and possible paralysis associated with spina bifida. There was a familiar thought on my part ("How far should I pursue the relationship between her fears and expectations?") even as Rebecca, clearly wanting to maintain her compo-sure, struggled to express her own guilt in words. At the time of her pregnancy she had been taking a medication known to increase the chances of fetal spina bifida.

While acknowledging the obvious risks, she still wanted to discuss her options for undergoing open-uterine fetal repair. When asked why she would want to take such risks, Rebecca said it was because she wanted to do what she could now to help make things better for her baby's future. Indeed, after the three-day counseling process, Rebecca decided to undergo open-uterine surgery on behalf of her child-to-be.

During that procedure, when Rebecca's fetus was positioned for neurosurgical repair of the spinal defect, the fetal heart rate decreased. After several attempts at repositioning, the surgeons decided to replace the fluid in the uterus and then wait to see if the heart rate recovered. After the appropriate length of time, they again attempted to reposition for surgical repair, which again resulted in decreased fetal heart rate. It was decided then to abandon the fetal repair and to close the incisions.

Rebecca's recovery, monitored in the standard fashion, seemed uneventful until later in that first day after surgery. Then there was an unforeseen outcome: absence of fetal heart tones. An ultrasound confirmed the fetus had died, but what caused the demise was unclear.

The next morning, after the fetus was retrieved, I went to see Rebecca and her mother. Her mother motioned me in. Obviously grieving, Rebecca was in her hospital bed. Then, during a set of compelling moments that I remain unable to describe adequately, Rebecca's mother gently unwrapped a blanket to show me the defect on the spine of this 23-week-old fetus.

Haunting aspects

The threats of injury, handicap, and disability – all manifest in the spinal lesion on the back of the tiny body that Rebecca's mother so tenderly showed me – were no longer limited to the vivid textures of that little body. Instead, I experienced a visceral sense of the struggle to understand their meaning. Yet, even that uncanny sense was suppressed by a more pervasive, equally subtle – and immediate – sense of astonishment: While that little body was dead, I was alive. The depth of my riddle in this experience was thus encompassed by what Nietzsche called the "profoundest problem in ethics": "How can anything pass away which has a right to be?"[9]

Strange, because immediately before – while observing the specific, complex, and compelling beauty of her mother's tenderness while unwrapping the blanket and presenting the fetus – I had not been able to think of anything. I was transfixed by the finely drawn profile of unfinished features and the almost translucent textures of that little face against the white blanket. Right there and then, that sense I would describe as the "uncanny" was sourced in the intimate and profound relation that is my self and my body, a relation in which it is equally true that my body – and hence my world – is experienced as strange and alien. Indeed, for each of us, as my teacher Zaner says, "this embodying organism is experienced by me as my exposure to things, ultimately as the locus of that most alien of all: my own death."[10]

I use this term "uncanny" to suggest the way that the quality of reassurance in the familiarity of regular activities carried out in clinical encounters is unlocked and transformed into "the strangest of the strange."[11] This experience consists in its sudden and radical departure from the familiar, with the ambiguous sense of "the other side of the mirror" that is not reflecting back. Thinking back on this experience with Rebecca and her mother, I am reminded of Zaner's teacher, Natanson, when he says, "The experience of the uncanny cannot be planned by the individual who is seized by what is primordially strange. The dread which often accompanies the uncanny is related to death, to the dead, and to the dying."[11] In being "seized by what is primordially strange," something emerges that may be crucial to what we are pointing to, and to what we mean, when we talk about moral experience.

The "something" that emerges is that, for most of us, it is not easy to look into our own sense of values inherent in the performance and activities of ethics consultations, especially when our *basis* for such values is challenged by the intimate experience of illness, injury, disability, and dying. Indeed, it is precisely at these times that we typically prefer to rely on the relative stability of those values that enable us to move forward, to continue to do what we do. But such participation presents its own hazards: In the experience of the uncanny, how do we distinguish *genuine* from *transiently perceived* beliefs and values? After all, in the reverse of the familiar there arises a sharp awareness of uncertainties and vulnerabilities brought about by the need to identify and then distinguish among genuine beliefs, especially in those situations where these may be most challenged.

That awareness institutes boundaries, and thus a sense of limitation, that underlie presumed responsibilities in ethics consultation.[12] The ethics consultant's own moral disruptions are not necessarily – and especially not in the most discrete, intimate, and possibly crucial ways – analogous to those of the others the consultant might want to help. Nonetheless, ethics consultants may be confronted with implications or insights into their own understanding – or misunderstanding – about those beliefs and values most cherished to themselves, and may be to others.

In other words, ingredient in the activities and familiarity of moral experience in ethics consultation is the individual's discovery of his/her humanity – and the fact that he or she lacks important and real knowledge about what that means. A dynamic and critical element of meaning in moral experience relies upon the idea that reflexivity is not merely stipulated in the self's own insularity. Rather, it occurs *in* the relationships and context of its life, *in* a body and world *it did not choose and it cannot create*.[10] One crucial sense of "moral," then, is encountered precisely in the dramatic shift of attention by a "self" to the latent vulnerabilities of embodiment, accident, and chance shared with other persons and evoked in the experience of the threatened, impaired, or dying other.

And so, thinking back on my encounter with Rebecca's and her mother's loss, I have a familiar question: What should I do or say about such strenuous riddles, with their hair-trigger emotional depth charges and their abysmal, agonizing outcomes? Was I, along with Rebecca and her mother, well advised to seek the path of reconciliation and acceptance? Rebecca, after all, would not now be burdened with the fuller extent of the personal, psychological, medical, and social challenges characteristic of spina bifida. And she had "done everything" available to her rather than "waiting to see" what resulted from standard treatment.

Professional reflections

Of course, these dimensions of human experience and their potential meanings are even more subtle, more intimate, harder to explain, and thus likely to yield potential criticisms of ethics consultation. There exists here a discernible tension between two concerns that relate directly to typical ethical norms. As an ethics consultant, I am confronted with the dual considerations of respect and harm in a mutual responsibility shared with the persons I am trying to help. Thinking about my involvement with Rebecca's situation illustrates a core question about responsibility, both *for me* as an ethics consultant as well as *in* my relationship with others: Is it more harmful or beneficial to identify and articulate crucial factors that remain unspoken, possibly unacknowledged, and perhaps unimagined?

The first point is obvious: What if those others – as is the tendency of many – would rather not examine themselves in that focus of tormented choices, despairing commitments, and furtive allegiances in their own lives? For example, surely it is dreadful that any child should have to live with serious and undeserved disabilities. Just as surely, that dreadful awareness is difficult to face, especially if a parent encounters dread in him or herself about the prospect of living with and caring for this child. What if, during discussions about the choice of maternal–fetal surgery, there are clues that a pregnant woman (or her partner) dreads the thought of caring for a disabled child, but she or he seems willing to leave that thought unaddressed? Should I, or anyone else, talk about that dread explicitly as an issue to be addressed? If the decision to have surgery is an elective one, what are the merits of raising for discussion (as I did with Rebecca and her mother) the idea that the motivation to have surgery might be more *against* disability than *for* the surgery?

The second and more complex point is this: If ethics consultants shy away from and do not articulate and rigorously examine such influential dispositions, values, and beliefs, then what is left of "ethics"? This is especially the case where the activities of clinical ethics consultation involve immersion in the uniqueness of actions, emotions, relationships, and circumstances of other persons' lives. That sort of immersion is certainly illustrated by such moments as when Rebecca's mother presented the stillborn fetus to me. Likewise, a similar sort of immersion occurred when, after I explicitly raised the idea that Rebecca's motivation to have the surgery might be as much against disability as for the surgery, she agreed, while crying, that hers might be such a motivation and then went on to say that she still wanted the surgery.

Clearly, such motivations raise other issues as well. For instance, obligations on the part of clinicians who might offer maternal–fetal surgery, while magnified by perceptions about fetal vulnerability, are compounded by the vulnerability of the woman upon whose life the fetus depends. If it makes sense to say that such vulnerabilities increase the clinicians' obligations, real questions persist regarding the view that authorization for the fetus as a clinical patient is derived primarily from respect for the woman's autonomy.[13] That view is perhaps most complicated regarding open-uterine surgery for a previable fetus with a nonlethal malformation like spina bifida. The point is this: The widely accepted and otherwise sound commitment to autonomy does not help much when discussions must focus on the contents that inform the justification of one choice rather than another. Reliance on "autonomy," of itself, won't address the choices women face, especially given the ways that their personal convictions preshape and preinterpret the very sense of such key notions as "alternative," "choice," "treatment option," even "decision," all of which make "informed consent" quite problematic.[1]

After all, in what ways could one explain to Rebecca and her mother the meaning of those concepts, whether prior to, or after, the death of Rebecca's fetus? To what extent might I have gone and to what degree of blunt and graphic language might I have used to explain to Rebecca and her mother that a very real part of the choices she faced was the possibility that she would be lying in a hospital bed grieving, with her dead fetus close by, wrapped in a blanket?

Finally, my point about responsibility is to raise this question: To what extent – if at all – does a woman freely deciding to have maternal–fetal surgery relieve those others involved (physicians, nurses, other family members, and so on) from responsibility for the consequences of the actions taken; in particular, those consequences that might reasonably be foreseen to cause harm to a fetus?[6] Does this pertain as well to the involved ethics consultants?

Outcome

Rebecca was discharged after three days and, in the usual course of events, the nurses and physicians did not discuss much about what had happened. They went on to other things and other patients. Although what caused the outcome of her case was still uncertain, it was folded into the practice of open-uterine surgery as one of the things to be avoided. Because the fetal repair was not achieved, and because the cause of the fetal demise was unclear, her outcome was an "outlier" to other published information, now obscured by years and personnel changes in the fetal-surgery team.

Still, the questions I have raised accompany me as I go to greet the next young couple, with their first pregnancy and a routine ultrasound at 18 weeks showing findings of spina bifida. They are curious about why they might be meeting someone called an ethics consultant and why they need to find out more about the randomized clinical trial in which they might decide to enroll.

There are, of course, always other questions: If I am haunted in these ways, does that warrant my saying that this surgery should not be pursued in my institution? If not, what would be the basis for such a warrant?

Discussion questions

1. In view of the complexity of issues regarding decision making, should ethics consultation become a standard part of the consultation process for innovative maternal–fetal interventions that increase the risk of fetal demise? How should the role of ethics consultation be explained in such a process?
2. To what degree should an ethics consultant's own trepidation or fortitude factor into the ways that prominent issues in a situation are evaluated and discussed? Can we identify indications that would signal when an ethics consultant's personal, moral reactions to a patient's predicament have distorted the consultation process?

3. What basis for evaluation would you use to determine whether it is more harmful or beneficial to explore difficult, even painful, aspects of a patient's life or values in the interest of the patient's long-term well-being? How would you know when to explore hidden values and when not to?
4. During discussions about the choice to have maternal–fetal surgery, there are clues that a pregnant woman dreads the thought of caring for a disabled child, but she seems willing to leave that difficult thought unaddressed: What are the merits of explicitly raising for discussion (as was done in this case with Rebecca and her mother) the idea that the motivation to have the surgery might be more *against* disability than *for* the surgery?

REFERENCES

1. Bliton MJ. Ethics: "Life before birth" and moral complexity in maternal-fetal surgery for spina bifida. *Clin Perinatol*, 2003; 30: 449–64.
2. Chervenak FA, McCullough LB. A comprehensive framework for fetal research and its application to fetal surgery for spina bifida. *Am J Obstet Gynecol*, 2002; 187(1): 10–14.
3. Lyerly AD, Mahowald MB. Maternal-fetal surgery for treatment of myelomeningocele. *Clin Perinatol*, 2003; 30: 155–65.
4. Bruner JP, Tulipan N. Intrauterine repair of spina bifida. *Clin Obstet Gynecol*, 2005; 48(4): 942–55.
5. *Management of Myelomeningocele Study (MOMS): A Randomized Trial of Prenatal Versus Postnatal Repair of Myelomeningocele.* The National Institute of Child Health and Human Development, Fetal Surgery Units Group, 2003.
6. Bliton MJ, Zaner RM. Over the cutting edge: How ethics consultation illuminates the moral complexity of open-uterine fetal repair of spina bifida and patients' decision making. *J Clin Ethics*, 2001; 12(4): 346–60.
7. Churchill LR, Bliton M, eds. Parental voices in maternal-fetal surgery. *Clin Obstet Gynecol*, 2005; 48(3): 509–607.
8. Doherty D, Shurtleff DB. Pediatric perspective on prenatal counseling for myelomeningocele. *Birth Defects Res A Clin Mol Teratol*, 2006; 76: 645–53.
9. Nietzsche F. *Philosophy in the Tragic Age of the Greeks.* Translated by M. Cowan. Washington, DC: Regnery Publishing, 1962 (reprinted 1996); 48.
10. Zaner RM. *The Context of Self: A Phenomenological Inquiry Using Medicine as a Clue.* Athens, OH: Ohio University Press, 1981; 52–5.
11. Natanson M. *The Erotic Bird: Phenomenology in Literature.* Princeton, NJ: Princeton University Press, 1998; 54, 133.
12. Bliton MJ, Finder SG. Traversing boundaries: Clinical ethics and moral experience in the withdrawal of life supports. *Theor Med Bioeth*, 2002; 23(3): 233–58.
13. Harris LH. Rethinking maternal-fetal conflict: Gender and equality in perinatal ethics. *Obstet Gynecol*, 2000; 96(5): 786–91.

Part II

The most vulnerable of us:
pediatrics

5

She was the life of the party

Douglas S. Diekema

Case narrative

"She has always been the life of the party," her mother responded when asked to describe her 7-year-old daughter. "She has always been at the center of everything in our household . . . she is so full of joy." Despite that description, Rachel's parents were asking the pediatric intensive care unit (PICU) team to withdraw the ventilator and vasopressors keeping Rachel alive.

I first met Rachel when she arrived at our hospital three days earlier in septic shock. I was the emergency department (ED) physician on duty when Rachel arrived by ambulance. Her blood pressure was lower than it should have been. She was cool and pale, her arms and legs mildly cyanotic, her frightened face partially hidden behind an oxygen mask. I gently lifted the mask and told her she would be OK and that we were going to take care of her. We quickly started IVs and antibiotics. Shortly after her arrival, one of our nurses noticed that Rachel had developed spots on her feet. On closer examination, they appeared to be petechiae (pinpoint-sized spots that represent bleeding into the skin), a sign that Rachel's illness might be the result of a microorganism named meningococcus. Meningococcus infections can progress rapidly and lead to death or serious complications. Rachel's blood pressure improved with our efforts, and I transferred her to the PICU. She still looked terrified as she was wheeled out of the emergency department. I took her hand, looked into her face, and told her once again that we would take good care of her.

With Rachel now in the hands of another team, I went back to seeing other patients in the busy emergency department, wondering occasionally throughout the day how she was doing. It was another busy day in the emergency department, and soon Rachel was forgotten.

Three days later I was on-call for ethics consultations when my beeper went off. My return call was answered by the PICU attending who said they wanted my help with a young patient. She was a 7-year-old with meningococcemia who had developed purpura fulminans, a life-threatening complication of the infection that results in widespread bleeding and tissue destruction. My hopes that Rachel was recovering were dashed. She now needed two vasopressors, a high-oscillation ventilator, and peritoneal dialysis.

Rachel's parents, who I had not previously met, were requesting that the ventilator and vasopressors be withdrawn and that Rachel be allowed to die. The PICU attending expressed several reservations about their decision. First, he and the rest of the team felt there were too many uncertainties surrounding Rachel's condition and prognosis; it seemed premature to withdraw life-sustaining treatment. He speculated she had a 50% chance of survival at best. She had suffered huge blood clots to all four extremities. "If she survives," he said, "she'll likely require bilateral above the knee amputations and bilateral arm amputations at the level of the elbows or forearms." The best-case scenario in the event of survival included dozens of reconstructive surgeries and a medicalized existence for years. Her neurologic outcome was unknown. Strokes were a strong possibility, but radiologic imaging of her brain was not possible given her present level of support. Despite that, most members of the team felt the decision to withdraw life-sustaining treatment was premature, especially without knowledge of whether she had suffered brain injury. Finally, the attending was concerned that the parents were making a decision based on the potential burden of future care and not because they felt it was in Rachel's best interest. This concern was fueled by the fact that while religion played a role in the decision, the decision did not seem to comport with the way others from a similar religious background had behaved in similar situations.

I walked to the PICU and entered Rachel's room. She was unrecognizable – bloated and purple, unresponsive amid the mass of high-tech equipment. I spent a long time talking with Rachel's parents. They described themselves as evangelical Christians who possessed a strong faith and regularly attended a church in their hometown. Rachel's mother had been the daughter of missionary parents, and the family had done missionary work overseas. Difficult decisions were not new to them, and they always tried to make the best of trying circumstances. One of Rachel's older siblings had been born with trisomy 21 (Down's syndrome). Rather than see this as a burden, Rachel's parents described him as a gift from God and an important member of their family, one of five children, each of whom played an important role: "We love him dearly, he's blessed our family immeasurably, and our family would not be the same without him."

Rachel's parents felt they had made a valiant, aggressive effort to save their daughter's life. They expressed gratitude toward everyone involved in her care, but they firmly conveyed their wish to cease aggressive treatment, including the ventilator and vasopressors. They knew this would almost certainly result in Rachel's death, but they were comfortable with that outcome. Her father argued that the team had struggled for three days to keep Rachel alive and there had been no sign of a positive response. It seemed clear that God was calling her home: "We don't believe that God requires us to pursue every aggressive means possible to bring our daughter through to what she will face on the other side. Everyone has made a valiant effort, but it is time to stop. If despite ceasing aggressive care she survives, we will praise God, take her home, love her and value her, regardless of what her handicaps might be. But we do not feel God requires us to pursue continued aggressive means to that end." Her mother added, "You have to understand that when you believe there is a wonderful life after death, you know your daughter will be going to a better place. Why should we use every technological means to forestall that possibility when it looks like God is calling her home?" They had discussed this decision with their entire extended family, their pastors, and many others within their church community. All had agreed that this was an acceptable decision.

I shared the medical team's discomfort with their request to withdraw life-sustaining treatment along with the team's sense that the decision seemed premature at this stage in Rachel's illness. In an effort to identify a compromise, I asked Rachel's parents if they would be willing to wait a few days before withdrawing the ventilator and vasopressors.

"We've made our decision and we would prefer not to wait any longer. We have already brought Rachel's brothers and sisters to the room to say goodbye. It is time to let her go." I expressed my concern that the medical team would certainly resist withdrawing the ventilator until Rachel could breathe on her own. Without allowing time for paralytic drugs to wear off, the team felt it would be contributing to Rachel's death. Rachel's father replied that they understood, they did not want the staff to experience any guilt over this decision, and they were willing to allow time for paralytic agents to wear off so that the team did not feel responsible in any way for her death. They were also willing to grant me a day to convene the ethics committee if I felt that was necessary.

As the ethics consultant in this case, I felt the parents were making an appropriate decision under tragic circumstances, but given the uncertainties in prognosis and the fact that all of the physicians and nurses caring for Rachel felt it was premature to withdraw life-sustaining treatment, I called a meeting of the full ethics committee. Given the controversy, it seemed wise to take advantage of the more intensive discussion and multiple perspectives of the full committee.

Professional reflections

During the ethics committee meeting that followed, members expressed the same concerns that had been verbalized by the PICU team. Nearly all members expressed discomfort with the decision the parents were making. They also expressed uneasiness about allowing the withdrawal of life-sustaining treatment when there was a reasonable likelihood of survival and concern about the reasons behind the parents' decision to change course. Why rush? Why not allow a few more days? It became clear that underlying most of the committee's concerns was a sense of unease concerning the parents' motives.

In situations involving acute events in otherwise healthy children, ethics committee members had come to expect parents to arrive at a place where they could accept withdrawal of life-sustaining treatment only after the medical team had reached that conclusion. Did the parents truly have Rachel's interests in mind or were they more concerned about the demands that would result from her survival? Interestingly, what made many committee members most uncomfortable was that the parents held religious views that seemed unusual because they did not correspond with the views of parents in similar PICU situations who professed to be evangelical Christians. In those cases, the experience of the ethics committee and PICU team had been that those parents would refuse to allow withdrawal of care, claiming that faith required them to "do everything possible" in the belief that God would perform a miracle if their faith was strong enough. Rachel's parents, by contrast, were asking to withdraw life-sustaining treatment even before the medical team was ready to recommend that course. Committee members seemed ready to conclude that either these parents were behaving irrationally, in a way inconsistent with their core beliefs, or they had other motives and were using their belief as a cover for those motives. It was these apparent contradictions rather than concern about the actual decision that seemed to plague the committee most.

As the only member who had met the family and who had discussed their views with them, it seemed clear to me that ethics committee members were seeing this case through the wrong set of lenses. That distorted vision was impairing the committee's ability to make a reasonable judgment. My role at that meeting became one of interpreter. I was able to assume this role because I had spent time with Rachel's family, but I also shared with the family a religious tradition.

Rachel's parents had told a very coherent story. The narrative they shared with me about their individual lives, their life as a family, their place in a religious community, and their understanding of the demands of their faith were all consistent with the decision they now wanted to make. When viewed within the family's narrative, the decision they sought to make had integrity. Committee members had difficulty with the family's decision because they were placing the decision within the context of a narrative they had created based on their experience with similar families. They had not seen the decision in the context of the family's own narrative, which was consistent with the views of the family's church and pastor.[1] It was easier for me to recognize this because I shared the family's religious tradition and I could see how their decision was consistent with that tradition.

Parental decisions need to be understood within the family's narrative, not our own. One strategy we often use to understand others is to identify features we think will help us understand them better. Knowing that someone is an evangelical Christian tells you something about him/her, but there are enormous variations in faith and belief from one evangelical to another. People are complicated, and they cannot often be placed in tidy categories. That is why narrative is important, and that is why it is important for medical providers to listen carefully to narratives.

In this case, the greatest concern of the medical team and the ethics committee was not the decision that Rachel's parents were making. Although many would have preferred to wait until a more certain prognosis had been established, nearly all agreed that the decision they wished to make was acceptable given the likelihood of survival and the significant burdens attached to that survival. Continued aggressive care might be acceptable and even desirable (in the minds of some), but it was not mandatory. Committee members had been most concerned with whether the parents' motives were proper. This question arose primarily because the committee did not feel the decision the parents were making was consistent with the decision an evangelical Christian would make.

Moral decisions are not simply abstract exercises. Narrative is necessary to understand who people are, what is important to them, and how they see the issue in question and the values at stake. Without that understanding, the decisions people make may seem arbitrary and incomprehensible. The motives of Rachel's parents could only be understood by listening to their story. Once we had done that, it was clear that our concerns were unfounded, and the committee agreed that the family's decision should be supported.

Haunting aspects

My memories of Rachel and her family are more vivid than any other patient with whom I have been involved. The case haunts me for several reasons. First, Rachel was my patient in the emergency department, and our first meeting took place under critical conditions. I felt good about the care we provided to her, but it haunts me that her disease progressed despite everything we had to offer. Every emergency department physician has patients who ultimately die, but Rachel affected me more than any other. The thing about Rachel that I will never forget is her frightened face looking into mine, so clearly asking for help. She was very much alive when I first met her, and her face was voicelessly pleading with me to help. When she left the ED, I thought we had been successful in reversing the course of her illness, and I attempted to reassure her by telling her she would be OK. It haunts me that I could not keep that promise.

Second, this was the only time in 15 years that I was asked to do an ethics consult for a patient I had cared for in the ED. I had nearly forgotten about that little girl when the call came, and it was disturbing to make the connection and realize that my hope that she would be OK had been shattered by this consult. The scared little girl I had last seen leaving the ED could not be the bloated, purple, unresponsive child I was now looking at in the PICU. The abrupt transformation that had occurred over those three days was jarring . . . and haunting. On the other hand, I felt no conflict between my previous role as Rachel's physician and my current role as ethics consultant. While I felt I understood her situation better because I had previously cared for her, I was no longer acting as her physician and I was no longer making clinical decisions. This allowed me to focus on the ethical issues.

Third, Rachel's parents were the most thoughtful, articulate, grounded parents I had ever met in such a tragic situation. They were also the most morally mature people I had met. It was as if they had assumed the role of caretaker for everyone in the hospital, and we had become the ones needing support. While they remained devoted to their daughter, rarely leaving her side, they also wanted everyone else to be at peace with the decision they were making. Although they were ready to switch the trajectory of Rachel's care, they allowed another day so the medical team could accept their decision. They wanted it to be clear that the responsibility for this decision was theirs and not the medical team's.

Finally, Rachel's family came from the same religious tradition that I did. We had much in common, and their beliefs mirrored my own. Rachel's parents soon recognized what we shared. They asked me, "What would you do if this was your daughter?" I had always struggled with how to answer that question for a parent, precisely because this was not my child and I could not possibly know how I would respond in a similar situation. But I also knew I had to answer the question. Rachel's parents needed an answer, not an attempt to dance around the question. At the same time, the question made this personal. I also had a young daughter. By asking the question, they forced me to share their situation in a way I had not before. Perhaps it was the family's way of inviting me to sit alongside them in this difficult time.

I answered as honestly as I could. I responded that I could not possibly know what I would do in such a horrible situation and that I hoped I would never find myself in a similar situation. I told them that my best guess was that I would not yet be ready to make the decision they were making and that I would need a little more time and the additional information that a few more days might bring. "But just because that's how I think I would respond in a similar situation does not mean that I think you are making the wrong decision for your daughter."

Outcome

Initially, most members of the ethics committee were uncomfortable with the decision being made by Rachel's parents and questioned their motives. These concerns were somewhat alleviated with a better understanding of how that decision fit within the family's narrative and a recognition that this decision was not at odds with the family's professed religious beliefs. In fact, I argued that Rachel's family had genuinely reflected upon and acted out their faith. Rachel's family believed that the final outcome was in God's hands and was not dependent on what they wanted. They truly left the final outcome in God's hands. They had acted as responsible agents in trying to keep Rachel alive with the tools available to them, but they were now willing to recognize that God might have other plans.

The committee could then focus on whether this was an acceptable decision for a parent to make given the medical circumstances. Generally, parents are allowed to make decisions about the health care of their children unless the decision places the child at significant risk of serious harm.[2] In this case, the ethics committee weighed Rachel's likely death after withdrawal of the ventilator and vasopressors against the odds that she would die even with aggressive treatment and the possibility of future disability, burden, and suffering if she survived. After an extensive discussion, the committee agreed that this decision fell below the ethical and legal thresholds for legal intervention to force continued therapy. The committee elected to support the parents' decision to withdraw the ventilator and vasopressors. Most members of the committee felt conflicted about this decision, a reflection of the tragic nature of the situation.

Rachel's parents agreed to give the PICU team another half-day to allow paralyzing agents to wear off. The ventilator was removed and vasopressors were stopped the day after the ethics committee meeting. Rachel died peacefully a short time later with her parents sitting beside her saying goodbye one last time.

Discussion questions

1. When parental decisions arise from cultural or religious beliefs, should the ethics committee judge those decisions differently than similar decisions that do not seem to arise from cultural or religious beliefs?
2. Should the motives of parents play a role in whether the decision they make on behalf of a child is acceptable?
3. Should parents be allowed to decide to withhold or withdraw life-sustaining treatment in cases where there are significant burdens attached to survival? What if those burdens accrue to caretakers rather than to the child?

REFERENCES

1. Charon R. *Narrative Medicine: Honoring the Stories of Illness*. New York: Oxford University Press, 2006.
2. Diekema DS. Parental refusals of medical treatment: The harm principle as threshold for state intervention. *Theor Med Bioeth*, 2004; 25(4): 243–64.

6

The sound of chains

Jeffrey Spike

Case narrative

It was an anomalous case from beginning to end. The request came from social work, which is not strange in and of itself. It was the nature of the request, rather than its source, that was unusual. Should the mother of a patient be allowed to visit her child? Of course, additional details followed: The child was a shaken baby, and the mother was a suspect. From my phone conversation I inferred that many people on the team felt the answer should be "No."

My gut reaction was that a mother should be allowed to visit her child unless there is solid evidence that it would endanger the child. Unfortunately, in this case, the harm had already been done. Furthermore, even if she were the one who had harmed the child, it was most likely due to a momentary loss of control – terrible yes, inexcusable yes, but unlikely to happen again in a controlled and supervised environment.

I try not to give my "gut" reaction over the phone. Sometimes I know it is a well-justified opinion, and a slew of articles come to mind that could serve as references for the eventual consult note. However, I reserve judgment until I know enough of the individual circumstances to know whether the references or paradigms influencing my opinion are appropriate to the case.

The situation became more complex and confusing than I realized after I talked to the social worker. The mother and her boyfriend said they were both at home, and each said that neither had harmed the baby. It appeared that one was the perpetrator and the other was willing to defend the perpetrator. They both were most likely lying, but no amount of effort by the police coaxed either to confess. Logically, it was an example of the prisoner's dilemma, a well-known paradox that philosophers learn in graduate school. Both persons will receive the lightest sentence if each refuses to confess.[1]

A version of this chapter was originally published in *The Journal of Clinical Ethics*, 16(3): 212–17.

As with any consult, I went to see the patient so I could establish my own opinion rather than base it on the reports of others. The baby's name was "Angel," which only made the story sadder with its intimation of a spiritual being living in a better, less violent world. Adding to the poignancy, Angel* looked peaceful lying there in the tiny bed. His eyes were closed, and he looked like he was sleeping. He had no marks on him, no scars, no bruises, nothing. He had beautiful color and the fat cheeks of a healthy, well-fed baby. In my memory – clearly false – he was smiling.

But, Angel was still ventilator-dependent and in a coma after two weeks, and the neurological prognosis was that either the coma would be permanent or the coma would lighten and Angel would emerge into a permanent vegetative state (PVS). Some neurologists use the phrase "awake but unaware" to describe PVS. I knew that many family members as well as patient caregivers find that to be an even worse outcome than being comatose: The baby would be equally unaware, but the sleep–wake cycles and eye movements can make people caring for the baby be plagued by doubts (and even nightmares) about whether the baby is suffering.

When I returned to the unit the next day, I realized that my initial assumption about the staff wanting to prevent the mother from seeing her baby was correct. Whatever reticence I heard over the phone from the head social worker was not present among the bedside staff, who were clearly angry. Some of the nurses were very attached to this beautiful little baby, and they were outraged at the mother who they thought should not be allowed to visit. It was impossible to tell whether this was to punish the mother or to protect the baby. The two motivations were mixed together in the emotional swirl. Those who even considered a visit an option did so only in the hope that it would make her finally confess.

Furthermore, as the prognosis began to sink in and be accepted, there was a feeling among many team members that the mother should let her baby die in peace, with the loving nursing staff by his side. The nurses saw themselves playing a maternal role, which may be a relic of nursing's traditional role. Preliminary reports from the jail were that the mother refused to withdraw life-sustaining treatment. This further angered the staff, who saw that as prolonging suffering or dying rather than as prolonging a life.

Of course, there were legal twists that brought a "Catch-22" to the case. If the mother allowed her baby to die, then the charge would become murder. So, to put it mildly, she did not have any incentive to make that decision. Even the best parents have trouble "letting go" of children. In this situation she had already lost her child, and any confession meant she would go to jail, or her boyfriend would, or both.

If, ultimately, the mother refused to withdraw life support, then Angel would need to be in a long-term care facility for the rest of his life. At the time, there were

---

* I have used his real name because this case was public, not just from being in the court system but also reported in the newspaper. And his name adds to the poignancy and haunting quality of the case.

no long-term-care ventilator beds for children in the 14-county metropolitan area. However, this was not why the staff felt it would be better to stop the ventilator. It was also not an issue of the financial cost to society. Had Angel's mother been able and interested in visiting him regularly, I believe they still would consider it cruel or inhumane to keep him alive. I speculate this was based on two independent feelings (and I choose that word deliberately). The first was the idea that the perception that such patients cannot be aware of anything is neurological *hubris*. If the experts are wrong about this then such a life would be so terrible that no one would wish to live that way. The second feeling is that, whether the patient is aware of it or not, the resulting life is really not a human life and is so undignified that no one would want to be preserved and treated by strangers in such a way.

The staff was still divided on whether the mother should be allowed to visit. The nurses who were willing to let the mother visit also wanted me to be there, with the hope that I could persuade her to stop life-sustaining treatment for the sake of the baby. But what could I say to persuade her to withdraw life-sustaining treatment? According to the best neurological knowledge, Angel was not suffering. Caregivers are the people most likely to suffer in cases involving patients in a PVS.

I wrote a short note and also explained to the social worker that I felt the mother should be allowed to visit. I stated that I would be willing to be present if that was what the doctor and the staff wanted. This short handwritten note did not provide justifications (that is saved for the final note, typewritten and researched), but my sense was that even if the mother were responsible for the injury, she no doubt deeply regretted it now, and there was no reason to further punish her by not allowing her to see Angel. That it also meant her seeing the consequences of the act could not be a reason to prevent her from seeing him; if anything, it would be better for her to make a decision based on a full understanding of his condition.

Once an ethics consultation is called, it is standard procedure for the ethics consultant to join family meetings. There are many reasons for this. First, the family should have a chance to meet and talk with every person involved in the process. Second, the ethics consultant can aid communication by making explicit some things that medical experts take for granted but that members of the family might not know. It is not unusual to go to a meeting unsure of whether I can add anything valuable only to find that I contributed an insight that would have been overlooked. The lesson is that there is no way to know *a priori* if my presence will be needed, and hence it should be done as part of the routine. But I also cautioned that the team should not expect me to be able to change Angel's mother's mind, though I thought it would be right for someone on the team to discuss Angel's prognosis with his mother when she visited.

As I typically do, I spoke to the attending by phone to make sure I understood all the essential clinical information in advance. He assured me that the injury was devastating and irreversible. I told him that I would be at the meeting planned for a few days hence. I assumed that he would be at the meeting as well. When I arrived, the meeting seemed to have already begun. A nurse, the social worker, the mother, and two police escorts were crowded into the small room, and all spoke in hushed whispers. I was surprised when I looked around the room: There was no doctor in the group. The mother was by Angel's bedside with the nurse on one side of her and one of the police escorts on the other.

The mother was dressed in the orange jumpsuit of the local prison. I had not thought about what she would look like, and the prison uniform surprised me. Much more disturbing was that she was in chains. One heavy chain connected to metal bands around her ankles, presumably so she could not run. A second heavy chain connected to metal bands around her wrists. A third connected the two chains together so she could not raise her arms much above her waist. Indeed, either due to their short length, or their weight, or the weight of her guilt, she could barely move. A slow shuffle was all I ever saw, and whenever she moved there was a sound of heavy chains.

At first I felt like an intruder because everyone was standing up, close together, and facing the bed. But when I introduced myself I quickly sensed that everyone there had been waiting for me. The mother had tears in her eyes and was whispering to her baby. To me, at that moment, my only feeling was of overwhelming tragedy, not anger.

The baby's mother mumbled something so quietly I could not hear her. But there seemed to be some discussion of what she had said. The social worker turned to me as if to ask what I thought. I had to ask what she had said, and he explained to me that she wanted to hold the baby. I did not think her request was a bioethical issue; yet, I often admonish other ethics consultants not to avoid difficult issues by saying they are not bioethical issues. All too often, an issue can be perceived in different ways, and it will only be handled fairly if everyone acknowledges they have a legitimate role in resolving it. Otherwise, too much authority will settle into the hands of one person willing to take control. Ethicists are there to help balance the equation, if nothing else. And, to have denied this woman her request seemed punitive, all the more so because there was no way to know if she would ever see her baby again. So I spoke up and said I thought she should be allowed to hold her baby, even though (I added) I did not really think that decision was mine to make.

To my surprise, after some whispering between the two police guards, one took out a key and unlocked the prisoner's handcuffs. The social worker helped pick up Angel and put him into his mother's arms, and she sat in a rocking chair and held him. She talked to him, no doubt hoping for a response. But she got none. There was still no doctor there, and it gradually began to dawn on me that nobody was waiting for a doctor to show up. The meeting had begun, and now this was "my meeting" to run.

I was becoming more aware of the continual surprise this case presented; it did not follow the usual rules. I felt that I had taken on the role of an agent in the drama and was less of an adjudicator than I typically am. This contributed to the case's haunting quality. No one had ever suggested to me that this would be my meeting to run. If they had, it was in language so polite and veiled that I had missed it entirely. I most certainly had never run a meeting that in effect was the first and last chance to discuss a grim prognosis, as it is called in the medical world.

I had to think on my feet, carefully choosing each word that needed to be said as I was saying it, internally deliberating in order to not exceed the limits of what I was saying. I wanted to be accurate, and I did not want to coerce her into a decision. I also did not want to pull any punches. This was a case in which there would be no other chances for the information to sink in or for her to return with questions. I told her that nearly a month had passed since the injury, and not a single note in the chart indicated hope of meaningful recovery. I explained what the alternatives were: Stop the ventilator and let Angel die in his sleep or continue his life indefinitely in a nursing home once one could be found. I told her that while the decision was hers to make, many people, including many of the people at the hospital taking care of her baby, felt that the kindest and most respectful thing to do would be to let Angel die in peace. I added that I had known parents who had made that choice, and no one condemned them for it; in fact, they had received understanding and empathy for their difficult decision. But, I also admitted, I had known other parents who chose not to stop life-sustaining treatment, and though their babies never improved, no one could condemn the parents for that decision either.

She listened to me but said nothing. After what felt like too short a time, the guards indicated that her time was up. She placed Angel back in his bed, thanked me, and said she needed time to think about the alternatives. That was the last time I saw her.

Professional reflections

To remain neutral in any differences between the team and the patient or family, ethics consultants should avoid being mistaken for members of the healthcare team. This is one of the reasons doctors are at an inherent disadvantage as ethics consultants. However, that does not mean ethics consultants can afford to be uninformed. To be able to "sit at the table" a negotiator must do his or her homework and know as much about the situation as any of the principals. When it comes to medical information, one need not know the same things as the attending physician, but one does need to know as much as the *ideal patient* should know before deciding whether to consent to or refuse treatment. This is required to make sure the information is provided in a fair way and to ensure the patient understands and appreciates the consequences of whatever decision he or she makes.

I am always careful to tell patients that I am a PhD and not an MD, and that I am not there to give them medical information or advice. But I add that I may be able to clarify some things for them, and even when I cannot answer their questions I may be able to help them ask the right questions of their doctors.[2] Although the ethicist is never the decision-maker (that may have been what some people on the team wanted), part of the legitimate role of the ethicist is to help the patient make medical choices through effective informed consent or refusal.

Haunting aspects

This is a case I will never forget. It was clear from the beginning that the case involved nothing but misery, and that no one else on the ethics consultation service wanted to get involved. It fell to me because I was the director of the service. I did not realize it at the time, but this contributed to the haunting aura of the case: It was one of those few cases that I had no choice but to perform.

Many people who hear of this case wonder why the mother was even considered a valid surrogate decision-maker for her child. Experience taught me that no court-appointed guardian in my region would ever withdraw life-sustaining medical treatment. Hence there was nothing to be gained by having one appointed. Then there were things that many people would say only in private: Paying for this level of care for years or decades would be a terrible strain on limited healthcare resources. Many people who could gain a lot from small services would suffer from cutbacks due to a single costly case like this one. One often senses that people who call for an ethics consult expect miracles: rectify an injustice, or at least call to task the people who created it. These unanswered questions and unspoken doubts contributed to the palpable sense of anger toward the mother and to the dissatisfaction toward the ethics consult that I felt from good and well-meaning people involved in this case.

Other cases haunt me still. But as I sort them out, I see that most of them haunt me because of the lack of support or even opposition from sources that one would hope would be allies of clinical ethics. But that is disillusionment with one's department of health, attorney general, or hospital counsel. It is not caused by the case *per se*, which could have been handled more humanely had others listened to good advice and put the patient's interests ahead of their own legal fears, financial interests, personal needs, political agenda, or religious beliefs. Some of these pressures were at play in Angel's case, but it was made more haunting by the sense of being trapped in a horrible situation, like Angel himself.

Some might want to call this a sense of futility, but that word is overused in bioethics. It is not the futility of the treatment that is haunting. I prefer to consider this case an example of the true meaning of tragedy. In Angel's case, there was no consolation and no redemption to be found for anyone.

Outcome

As expected, the mother did not choose to stop life support for Angel. In this story, the mysteries were never solved. I doubt we will ever know who committed this horrible crime, which only adds to the case's reverberations.

Discussion questions

1. What role should your "gut reaction" have in an ethical analysis?
2. Is it better to keep a child alive but in a persistent vegetative state for 50 years than to let him die? Why or why not?
3. Do court-appointed guardians ever "pull the plug" where you work? Does this have a good ethical basis? If not, what might be done to change that?
4. Is it the ethicist's job to balance the power relations by making sure no one person drives the decision? Why or why not?
5. In certain cases, you may conclude that you must defend someone who is widely viewed as unethical. Will you be able to empathize with such a person? Should it matter to you if your colleagues revile the result you helped to accomplish?

REFERENCES

1. Sainsbury RM. *Paradoxes*, 2nd ed. Cambridge: Cambridge University Press, 1995, or Rescher N. *Paradoxes: Their Roots, Range, and Resolution*. Peru, IL: Open Court Press, 2001.
2. Spike JP. Assessment of decision making capacity. *Reichel's Care of the Elderly*, 6th ed. Philadelphia: Lippincott Williams and Wilkins, 2007; chapter 49.

7

Susie's voice

Rosa Lynn Pinkus, Stella L. Smetanka, and Nathan A. Kottkamp

Case narrative

Late one summer, a 9-year-old girl, Susie, complained of a headache and sore throat. Her parents took her to the pediatrician, who diagnosed her with strep throat and swimmer's ear and prescribed an antibiotic. Several days later, Susie was taken back to the doctor because the earache persisted. When she developed a dangerously high fever, her parents took her to a local emergency room where she was diagnosed with mastoiditis. To treat this condition, two intravenous anti-infection drugs were administered and a drainage wick was placed in her ear. She was then transported to the children's hospital for further evaluation. This was one week after her initial visit to her pediatrician. The evaluation at the children's hospital documented that Susie had been nauseated and had experienced night sweats and pain in her lower extremities. She had frequent bruises on her legs and was lethargic. A physical exam uncovered tender swelling around her right ear, and a complete battery of blood tests revealed T-cell acute lymphoblastic leukemia (ALL).

After Susie was diagnosed, her parents consented to chemotherapy treatment following the National Childhood Cancer Foundation CCG Protocol 1952,[1] part of an ongoing pediatric oncology treatment study. The study was designed to test the benefits of substituting certain medications from previous CCG protocols and of administering a triple rather than single intrathecal therapy (injecting chemotherapy directly into the cerebrospinal fluid using lumbar puncture). The study is also designed to measure relapse rates. Based on national averages, Susie's chance of cure was approximately 85%. Thirty years ago, the median survival for ALL was three to six months. Currently, 60% of patients survive 5 years or longer with greater numbers of long-term survivors or total cures. The attending oncologist told Susie's family that most children experience remission by the second week of chemotherapy treatment.[2] He advised the family that Susie would probably experience hair loss as a side effect.

When Susie began induction treatment, her blood count remained dangerously low. The oncologist intensified the treatment and Susie experienced nearly every possible side effect: vomiting, nausea, diarrhea, severe mouth blisters (both on the inside and outside of her mouth), sores throughout her gastrointestinal tract, blood poisoning, blood clotting, diabetes, yeast infections, severe headaches, leg cramps, bone pain, herpes, staph infections, E. coli infections, and severe pain and suffering. Eventually she required a morphine drip for the pain, and she took only liquid nutrition for three months. Her parents took Susie home to care for her, but she had to be readmitted to the hospital several times. After 93 excruciating days, Susie finally experienced full remission of the leukemia. Her protocol required two years of high-dose maintenance chemotherapy as a follow-up.

Once in remission, Susie traveled with her family to visit friends in California, against the advice of the attending oncologist. During the trip, she became very ill and developed a blood infection. Upon her return, the oncologist recommended a bone marrow transplant. However, no one in her family could provide matching bone marrow. At this point, the oncologist reduced the chance of cure with chemotherapy to 20–50%.

Given this new prognosis, Susie's parents met with the oncologist to discuss treatment options. They insisted later that the physician offered them three choices for their daughter's care: low-dose chemotherapy, high-dose chemotherapy, or forgoing any further chemotherapy. Susie and her parents had been told previously that low-dose chemotherapy would probably not be very effective. They knew that high-dose chemotherapy came with intolerable side effects even though it had brought Susie to remission.

Susie told her parents on many occasions that she would rather die than be subjected to additional chemotherapy and that she was willing to "go with Jesus." Her parents had lost faith in the experimental treatment and were convinced that she would die even after suffering side effects. After an agonizing week they told the oncologist that they and Susie had decided to forgo treatment.

Upon hearing this, the oncologist denied giving the family this third option. He now asserted that in his opinion, not treating Susie according to the protocol was tantamount to child abuse in the terms of the Child Protective Services statute.[3] He also felt that it exposed him to a medical malpractice suit should the parents reconsider. The parents and Susie remained steadfast in their decision. They perceived the physician as backing down on his word. He decided, in the face of the family's intransigence, that he was morally and legally bound to report Susie's parents to the Child Protective Services agency for medical neglect. By the terms of this statute, parental decision-making could be removed and given to a court-appointed guardian. Knowing that the family could not afford to pay a lawyer, the hospital social worker advised the parents to call the University Health Law Clinic, which is located within walking distance of the hospital. It provides free legal assistance from an attorney and law students. It was at this point that the social worker and the legal team set an ethics consult in motion.

Professional reflections

At the time this consult was placed, I (RLP) was one of six Center for Bioethics and Health Law ethics consultants working within the university hospital network. The center's consultation service follows a medical model. Consultants each carry a beeper and take calls two months of the year. The service is available 365 days per year, 24 hours a day. I had been involved in well over 70 cases at the time, and I often consulted the hospital legal counsel to get an opinion about the facts of a case. I had never been consulted by a lawyer, however, to take part in a case that had gone to legal counsel. "What," I asked the lawyer, "could an ethicist add?" The clinic's supervising attorney (SS, a coauthor of this case study) explained that from a legal perspective, she and the clinic law students would act as the parents' advocates, but she perceived that the problem needed both protection of the law and the sensitivities of bioethics. She placed a formal ethics consult with the intent of having the bioethicist act as a resource for both the legal team and the family. The law clinic felt that the bioethicist would provide a certain *entree* to the doctor and to the hospital and could also help promote communication between the oncologist and the family to avoid a lengthy and costly court battle. Hearing this, I agreed to accept the consult, and both the lawyer and I discussed with the family the option of meeting at the hospital with the oncologist. They accepted and the meeting was set.

As preparation for the meeting, I reread four cases involving adolescent and teenage patients in Baruch Brody's book *Life and Death Decision Making*.[4] Two were particularly relevant to the case at hand. The first involved an 11-year-old boy diagnosed and treated for ALL whose initial remission lasted only a year. He therefore carried a "dismal prognosis." Nevertheless, he continued treatment for another year and several remissions were accomplished. Each one involved increasingly severe side effects and a shorter time frame of recovery. The boy, now 13, relapsed and wanted another course of chemotherapy. His parents did not. Brody relates that the parents were given every encouragement in the initial induction and in subsequent ones as well. He suggests to physicians that there is wisdom in being realistic early on with patients when there is potential for a grim prognosis. How would Susie's case have progressed had the reality of side effects been appreciated prior to the initial course of chemotherapy?

The second case was that of "K," a 12-year-old boy treated over a three-year time frame for nasopharengeal carcinoma. Despite local radiation, chemotherapy, radical neck surgery, and chemotherapy, "K"s symptoms returned after his 15th birthday and he refused further treatment. The side effects, he reasoned, were not worth it. His parents wanted the physicians to continue. Brody described the boy's decision as a "realistic assessment." He also discussed the case within the frame of experimental therapy, where the assent of those being experimented on should be secured, especially when there is a potential for considerable suffering. As it had countless times before, Brody's impeccable logic and supportive tone became companions for me in this consult.

Because of the legal context, I was entering unchartered territory. In hindsight, I served as a "mediator," a role now recognized as one an ethics consultant should cultivate.[5] As I spoke with the social worker, the oncologist, Susie and her parents, and as I read the chart, their stories compelled me to ask: "Who speaks for this child? What is 'best' for Susie? Should her voice count? If so, how much?"[6] I wanted to discern the deep values and commitments of those involved, but sides had already been taken; positions were firm. My role was to provide some "space" for the family and the physician to resume a discussion – to re-explore the decision to take this matter to a judge.

Susie's parents, the oncologist, the hospital social worker, and the parents' lawyer met in a hospital conference room and I mediated the discussion. I cautiously repeated the facts as I understood them and watched for reactions. I repeated the reason for the meeting: to provide them with a chance to revisit taking a legal route to resolve this issue. Each day was important because if Susie experienced a relapse, no chemotherapy could be instituted. It would be too late. The oncologist was the first to speak. He denied giving the parents the option to discontinue treatment. Susie's mother countered that he had. I knew that we would never be able to re-create that conversation and simply said this. I remembered that they had both told me highly complimentary things about each other. The family respected the physician and was grateful for the care he had provided. The physician admired Susie and her parents for the way they fought and dealt with the ordeal of chemotherapy. Could they not get back to that point? At first they would not even look at each other. Eventually, my choice of words, my inflection of voice, caused someone in the family to laugh. That relieved the tension, and they finally began to discuss the best course of action.

The conversation ended with both parties agreeing to let a court decide whether Susie should have the chemotherapy treatments. My goal was to again focus the discussion on "what was best" for Susie, to encourage the parents and the oncologist to re-explore their positions and perhaps resolve the issue within the traditional doctor/patient relationship. There was an airing from both sides, but the conclusion was a resolve to move ahead as planned. The physician secured a lawyer from the hospital to represent him and my role as mediator continued. I was the only one now who could speak directly to both the physician and the family.

After that meeting, the legal team prepared a "Complaint in Declaratory Judgment" and "Motion to File Complaint Under Seal," which would allow the court to proceed without exposing either party to public scrutiny. There was very little precedent in our jurisdiction on the application of the statute's medical neglect provisions to parents' rights to discontinue medical treatment for terminally ill children. The Supreme Court had said that "[P]arents may be free to become martyrs themselves. But it does not follow they are free . . . to make martyrs of their children."[7] However, meeting only the highest standard of proof will permit parents' rights to be terminated. When the parents came to the legal clinic to sign their affidavits and to have them notarized, Susie's father spoke first and expressed his apprehension about going to court. He feared that a judge might consider chemotherapy Susie's only chance of cure, albeit small, and he worried that their case could somehow bring them unwanted publicity. The father then spoke on behalf of his family and indicated a change of plans. They wanted to start chemotherapy at a very low dose, with greater intensity achieved in steps. This was one of the other three options mentioned by the oncologist.

Several days passed before another meeting took place. The oncologist feared the parents' change of heart could be construed as a "coerced choice." He eventually agreed to meet and to provide Susie with the chemotherapy. He assured the parents that if Susie experienced the same harmful side effects as she had during the first regimen, he would use a less potent drug. In his words, "when toxicity was reached" he would take this measure. The mother asked pointedly, "Who gets to decide when toxicity is reached?" She wanted to assess this threshold and to allow Susie to decide when she could not handle the treatments any longer. I remember thinking "That's exactly right!" It made perfect sense to have a shared decision-making process here. This concept, which Susie's mother tacitly understood, provided a resolution to a potential impasse because it gave both parties influence. The resolution involved both lawyers drafting what would become a formal informed consent document that included a provision that treatment could be stopped at any time upon the parents' request. The oncologist felt legally protected by this document and the family was assured of a voice in Susie's treatment.

From the first meeting until the signing of this informed consent agreement, both the lawyer and I heard a constant plea from Susie's mother not to lose sight of the fact that her daughter's well-being was the reason for the whole confrontation. She continually expressed her concern that Susie be heard. We set up two meetings to give Susie a chance to talk about how she felt and what she wanted. She appeared in the small clinic class of law students with a psychologist skilled in discussing death and dying issues with children. She met with the legal team and me in our offices to let us hear her side. Susie's experience of death came through her grandmother's passing and through the death of certain pets. Her experience of suffering came through her grueling months of chemotherapy. She spoke of heaven as a beautiful place where she would see her grandmother again and, of course, Jesus and Mary.

Haunting aspects

We did not know until a few years after Susie's death how unsatisfying the resolution was to Susie's mother. The law clinic supervising attorney, who had become close with the family during the consult, met with Susie's mother to see how she was doing. The mother said her only regret was that she did not let Susie tell her side of the story to a judge. This statement jarred both of us. We relived how the events unfolded. Brutally honest with each other, we discussed whether our shared opinion that an out-of-court settlement would be best influenced the family's decision. We returned to the father's comments about not wanting to risk an adverse decision. The lawyer reflects: "If we had spoken with more confidence that the case could have been won, and if indeed the case had been won in court, would the mother calmly now look back on that day in court when Susie would have told her story to the judge?"[8] But Susie would still be gone, perhaps sooner. Was it the agreement that perhaps let Susie live a little longer? She had approximately six months of low-dose chemotherapy before she achieved toxicity. The chemotherapy was stopped and she relapsed. When asked this question, the mother only said it made no difference.

I go back to the difference between being a "mediator" and being an "ethics consultant" in this case. Susie and her family had bonded with their legal team. As "first responders" in a time of crisis, the team had provided relief. The lawyer, in particular, became a trusted friend throughout the case. She explains: "I took my son, who was the same age as Susie, to her 11th birthday party; I visited Susie a few days before she died; I paid my respects at the funeral home; I call the mother once in a while to see how they are doing. I would like to hear the mother say that she was satisfied that the case was resolved in the best possible way. But I don't think I ever will. Our personal mutual affection for each other does not change the way the mother feels. This haunts me."

I was perceived, rightly or wrongly, as an "outsider," connected in some way to the hospital, which was also perceived as the "enemy." What I felt during the consult was the family's fear and inability to trust me. I could not find a right way to approach Susie's mother and deferred to the lawyer on all counts. Given the adversarial construction of a legal framework, I think the family expected me to choose sides. If I was not for them then I must have been against them. My own fears were that during this time of indecision Susie would relapse, but I never shared my thoughts on these matters. This distance, at the time, was distressing to me. For years I would look back at this case, compare it to others I had been involved with, and wonder if the distance had somehow compromised the case.

Outcome

Approximately 7 months after the new regimen of chemotherapy began, Susie was back in the hospital intensive-care unit with life-threatening infections. Her original oncologist had moved to another city, and another physician in his practice had taken over Susie's care. He conferred with the parents during the September hospitalization, and all agreed to forgo any further treatment. It was as smooth as that. Susie was removed from chemotherapy treatment and continued to feel well.

She celebrated her 11th birthday, but by March she had relapsed. She died at home later that month.

Discussion questions

1. Should the ethicist have gotten involved in this consult? There are consults in which a legal recourse is probably the best option. Do you think this was one of those cases? Why or why not?
2. It is not common practice to revisit a consultation years after it has occurred to discern from the family its assessment of the process. In fact, it was the lawyer, not the ethicist, who did this. Should we routinely follow up on our consultations?
3. How should we "count" or interpret Susie's mother's "regret"?

REFERENCES

1. National Childhood Cancer Foundation, CCG Protocol: 1952. Available at http://www.nccf.org/nddf/protocol/1952.HTM. Accessed April 9, 1999.
2. Katz ER, Jay SM. Psychological aspects of cancer in children, adolescents, and their families. *Clin Psychol Rev*, 1984; 4: 525.
3. Child Protective Services Law, 23 Pa. C.S.A. § 6301, et. seq., 2001.
4. Brody B. *Life and Death Decision Making*. New York: Oxford University Press, 1988; 221–30.
5. Dubler NN, Liebman CB. *Bioethics Mediation: A Guide to Shaping Shared Solutions*. New York: United Hospital Fund, 2004.
6. Griffith DB. The best interest standard: A comparison of the state parens patriae authority and judicial oversight in best interest determinations for children and incompetent patients. *Issues Law Med*, 1991; 7:283, 300.
7. *Prince v Massachusetts*, 321 U.S. 158, 170 (1944), 170.
8. Evans J. Are children competent to make decisions about their own deaths? *Behav Sci Law*, 1995; 13: 27–41.

Access to an infant's family

D. Micah Hester

Narrative backstory

Before I arrived at my new institution, Baby Mo had been admitted at 6 weeks of age having endured an anoxic event of uncertain origin. Some speculated that his mom may have rolled over on him while sleeping, but nothing definitive was decided. This uncertainty led staff to speculate about the cause and the psychological motivations of the mother. The hypoxia was neurologically devastating, and the critical-care physicians initially believed Baby Mo would progress to brain death quickly. However, this did not occur. Although the physicians recommended "comfort care," aggressive therapy was continued at the parents' insistence.

As care progressed, Baby Mo was stabilized to the point that eventual home care on a ventilator was foreseeable. In order to provide this long-term ventilation, a tracheostomy (trach) was required. The parents, who wanted Baby Mo to go home with them, did not want a trach. The clinical staff saw this stance as inconsistent and medically and ethically unwarranted because long-term ventilation could not be adequately performed without the trach. If long-term care was desired, then the staff simply could not have its hands tied in trying to provide optimal care. At the same time, staff members noted the irony of pushing for an invasive procedure for a patient who they believed should be allowed to die peacefully, without aggressive treatment.

This was the first time an ethics consult was called concerning Baby Mo. Again, this occurred before my employment when ethics consults were handled exclusively by the hospital ethics committee. The clinical staff and ethics committee agreed that given the desires expressed by the parents, and the needs of Baby Mo, a trach was a medical and ethical requirement. The issue was taken to court, and literally moments before the Department of Human Services was to take custody of Baby Mo, the parents relented and allowed the trach to occur. Though Baby Mo remained in the chronic pulmonary unit for several more months, eventually he went home with his parents.

Case narrative

Fourteen months later I receive a call from a social worker in the pediatric intensive care unit (PICU). I had not met this woman since arriving eight months before. She asks if I am available to meet the following week to discuss a difficult case. She provides only a few details, but I gather that there is a young child in the PICU who has severe neurological damage, and the care team is frustrated with the care plan insisted upon by the parents. During that week, I hear a few more bits and pieces from one of the critical-care physicians, but I have nothing but a vague picture before I arrive for the meeting.

When I arrive at the designated conference room, several people are already there. As I open the door, one of them, whom I know from the ethics committee, pops up and catches me. "Micah," she says softly, "I guess you're here for the *next* meeting." Her inflection indicates her knowledge of the subject matter. "This is an administrative meeting for something else. We'll be done in a minute. Just wait outside until then, OK?" I agree, but while waiting outside I am aware of that "fish out of water" feeling welling up – that awkward "Wow, you can't tell the difference between meetings?" sense that reminds me that I know so few people that I cannot recognize who is and who is not part of the PICU staff. Once the meeting breaks up I am invited in. Quickly the room fills with faces I do not recognize except for a critical-care physician I met when interviewing for the job almost a year earlier. The family is not present.

In large group meetings called by others, I tend not to talk unless asked (or unless a particular point truly confuses my ability to analyze the situation). This has the benefit of allowing me to reflect on the situation without making premature pronouncements or insights. It has the detrimental consequence of creating expectations regarding my statements. When the ethicist speaks for the first time some 30 minutes into a discussion, people might expect my reflection to be insightful or profound.

During the meeting, discussion focuses on whether the care provided is, in fact, harming Baby Mo. The descriptions of the profound neurological devastation and the dramatic reflexes of Baby Mo whenever he is touched are very wrenching. Everyone on the team who is in the room agrees that Baby Mo is not well served by continuing the aggressive treatment. However, they also agree that the parents, who describe Baby Mo as having purposive actions, will not allow life-sustaining treatment to be removed. Superimposed on this is important recent history. Baby Mo was living at home on a ventilator with home nursing for a few weeks. During that time, his parents began to get frustrated by the home nurses. The parents were also frustrating the home nurses. Eventually, the parents would not allow the nurses into the home. Within two weeks, Baby Mo was fully septic and was brought to a local emergency room (ER) and transferred to our hospital (the sepsis resulted in a loss of fingertips). Once Baby Mo was admitted, the home ventilator company went to retrieve its equipment from the home but was not allowed to do so by a relative who lived there. This resulted in the home ventilator company's decision not to provide any further equipment to Baby Mo's parents.

Through this, and even though the parents proved to be ill-equipped during this episode at home, no one believed the parents to be anything but well intentioned. This fact, along with our chief counsel's and outside counsels' reading of state law, made any claim of legal negligence almost impossible. Ultimately, the decision was made to continue to follow the parents' wishes and hope that some event would significantly change the course of Baby Mo's care.

The facts of the case are numerous, and there are many more that could be provided – stories about religious beliefs not clearly tied to any systematic approach, exasperated friends who once tried to facilitate communication but no longer would, and numerous meetings of the hospital ethics committee, PICU staff, pulmonology unit, administration, and others. Baby Mo's second admission lasted over 12 months but eventually resulted in a new home ventilator company agreeing to provide equipment under specific conditions and Baby Mo (as of this writing) still residing at home with his parents.

Professional reflections

In many ways, this was a fairly "traditional" ethics case in the care of severely impaired infants.[1,2] The situation pitted differing accounts of what was best for Baby Mo – seemingly a struggle over "best interests." Yet parental authority was also in question.[3,4,5] The conflict was of vital importance because the decision was literally life-and-death. Stakes were acutely felt, and the experience of medical professionals was placed over and against the beliefs and desires of the parents. Even to this day, the positions seem quite intractable. Yet a careful and systematic consideration of the goals of care according to the parents, on the one hand, and the healthcare professionals, on the other, was only pursued through the "side door" of regular but indirect conversations.

In fact, one line of questioning I pursued with the attending physicians was to ask what they understood the goals of care to be *according to the parents*. The answers were speculative, though confident: "They want Baby Mo to go home." Why? "They believe a miracle will occur, and space (in our hearts and through our efforts) needs to be provided to let that happen."

In educational forums for both fellows and attendings in the PICU, I urged versions of the following questions to be pursued:

What are the goals of care according to the patient(family)?
> Why do they hold the goals they do?

Given their expressed interests and goals, what means (if any) are available and appropriate?
> Are there significant barriers to achieving the goals?
> Of the conflicts identified, are any intractable?

Are there more reasonable goals for the patient/family to have (that is, should their goals be redirected)?

Why are they more reasonable given what you have learned about the condition and prognosis of the patient and about the interests and goals of the patient/family?

What are the appropriate means of achieving these "more reasonable" goals?

These questions focus on the interest of the family (or patient if he/she can speak for him/herself). They attempt to provide material to construct a narrative of the family's interests robust enough to find common ground with the healthcare professionals. It is a participatory model, not simply one of bare autonomy and beneficence but of connection and cooperation.[6]

Haunting aspects

At times, hauntings are portrayed as the presence and actions of evil spirits, but hauntings can also take the form of voices speaking to us, as warnings, as reminders; they can beg and plead. Hauntings are often presented as externally manifest, but they just as often find form as internal, persistent, nagging dialog. Hauntings are typically described as something that is feared, but it seems plausible to see them also as stimulants for reflection and concern, a reminder to be humble and to be a catalyst for intelligent deliberation. What haunts me about the case of Baby Mo is that I cannot say whether a comprehensive attempt at robust conversation and deep insight into the parents' issues ever truly occurred. I suspect that to some degree it did. Why I suspect this says more about my deference to the goodwill of the physicians, nurses, and social workers with whom I work than it says about what I can attest to firsthand. This also haunts me.

With my PhD, in hand I have worked full time in a medical school for more than 9 years, and I have been available for ethics consultations since the first day. Having said this, I do relatively few consultations. While I have tools at my disposal to address a range of ethical issues in the clinic, the reality is that with my experiences being so small in number, I remain, at least in my own mind, a neophyte. The case I describe above still haunts me, and it came within the first year after moving to a new job. This haunting is persistent. It is a reminder of my inability to act when my insecurities dominate. I am haunted by the thought that I did not do enough, groped around too much, did not speak up, asked the wrong questions, and failed to push for further and deeper clarification.

The complications of the case can themselves be haunting. There is the difficulty of weeding through speculation to find which perceptions best clarify the overall picture and which simply muddy it. But through all this, my greatest error became more pronounced to me, yet I seemed unable to motivate myself to overcome it – *I had never heard from the family directly*. Each and every account of the situation came to me from a member of the hospital staff – a physician, a nurse, a social worker, a chaplain, a lawyer, even an administrator. While I tried to remain objective about the accounts I was getting, I failed to get an account from the parents themselves.

At first my rationale was simple: No one had asked me to speak with the parents. As I noted, I was first brought into this in the context of a team meeting about Baby Mo. I took my role to be additive, maybe elucidative, but not consultative, per se. Thus, I told myself that it was overstepping my role to request to meet the parents. As time went on and I was called into other meetings about Baby Mo, I began to tell myself that it was too late, that I was in "too deep" to ask now.

Clearly, both rationales were not well founded. Reasonable ethical insight must be based on a thorough deliberative process.[6,7,8] The omission of the parents' central narrative makes the deliberation suspect at best.[9,10] Also, two other personal factors played too great a role: a desire to be seen as helpful and a desire not to look foolish.

In a hospital, co-opting of bioethicists by the institutions of medicine can manifest itself in a number of ways. In this case, my concern not to be seen as anything but helpful by those who "invited" me was far too great. It remains a persistent problem of mine – the sense that to be viable in the hospital I must bring insight every time, I must be practical every time, and I must not offend or overstep my "expected" role every time. Further, as discussions drag on for minutes, hours, even days and weeks, it can be difficult to admit ignorance. In this relatively new environment, I was uncomfortable saying that I did not have all I needed to think well about these matters. This omission was significant.

I remain in awe of those who demonstrate comfort during ethical consultations. To this day, I aim to provide the best ethical deliberations and determinations I can without prejudicing *a priori* either the perspective of my medical colleagues or of the patients and families. I believe that thorough investigation into those perspectives will help yield the best outcomes. And yet, the case of Baby Mo and the flaws that haunt me are now there for anyone to read. They remain as persistent reminders of my responsibilities to gather information about and thoroughly reflect on the situations posed to me. I am also reminded not only of my foolish hubris but also of the need to speak out of ignorance to gather the necessary information and to understand as fully as possible the complexities of a case.

Outcome

As I mentioned above, Baby Mo remained in the hospital for many months. Occasionally, some mention of his status would find its way to me. Just before Baby Mo was discharged to home for the last time, his attending pulmonologist called to ask what I thought of his approach to the parents and Baby Mo. More openness seemed to be occurring between the staff and the parents. I had little to add, and Baby Mo, as I said, now resides at home. The staff remains a bit dissatisfied but accepting. The parents? I can only say that all secondhand and thirdhand accounts are that they are willing to abide by the arrangements made upon discharge – arrangements developed through nothing I did or said, but with my vague after-the-fact knowledge.

Discussion questions

1. To what degree do you feel comfortable when consulting? What situations, problems, people, or places create a reasonable level of comfort or problematic level of discomfort in any particular case?
2. Are you aware of the influences of being part of an institution that you are asked to evaluate? In what ways does your relationship to the institution and the staff affect your consultation practices and attitudes toward problems that arise?
3. Must every consultation include patients or families? Is it possible to provide useful ethical insight without hearing from all parties in every case?

REFERENCES

1. Munson R. *Intervention and Reflection: Basic Issues in Medical Ethics*, 5th ed. Belmont, CA: Wadsworth, 1996; 114–15.
2. McAliley LG, Daily BG. Baby Grace. *Hastings Cent Rep*, 2002; 32(1): 12–15.
3. Buchanan A, Brock D. *Deciding for Others: The Ethics of Surrogate Decision Making.* New York: Oxford University Press, 1984.
4. Ross LF. *Children, Families, and Health Care Decision Making.* New York: Oxford University Press, 1998.
5. Miller R. *Children, Ethics, & Modern Medicine.* Bloomington, IL: Indiana University Press, 2003.
6. Hester DM. *Community as Healing: Pragmatist Ethics in Medical Encounters.* Lanham, MD: Rowman & Littlefield, 2001.
7. Dewey J. *How We Think.* Boston: Heath & Co., 1910.
8. Dewey J. *Logic: The Theory of Inquiry.* New York: Henry Holt & Co., 1938.
9. LaPuma J., Schiedermayer DL. The clinical ethicist at the bedside. *Theor Med*, 1991; 12(2): 141–9.
10. Fletcher J. Ethics committees and due process. *Law Med Health Care*, 1992; 20(4): 291–3.

Part III

Diversity of desires and limits of liberty: psychiatric and psychological issues

Helping staff help a "hateful" patient: the case of TJ

Joy D. Skeel and Kristi S. Williams

Case narrative

"Ted Jacob," or "TJ," was a patient who, we quickly learned, tested the ethical resilience of most of the health professionals who worked with him.* He expanded our awareness of the types of conflicts that can be generated among the principles of nonmaleficence, beneficence, respect for persons, and autonomy.

TJ was 36 years old when the attending psychiatrist (KSW) on the consultation–liaison (C-L) psychiatry service first saw him. Both authors had heard about TJ from numerous health professionals because of the enormous problems he created on each admission. TJ, diagnosed with borderline personality disorder (BPD), characterized by intense emotional relationships, frequent crises resulting in suicidal ideation, and impulsive behavior, had been physically and sexually abused by his adoptive mother and ignored by an emotionally unavailable father. Beginning at age 11, he had numerous psychiatric admissions for attempted suicide and polysubstance abuse. His longest period of sobriety was during a marriage that lasted several years. TJ attended college for three years and majored in psychology. By history, he was bisexual, although his only known homosexual relationship was with his sponsor from Alcoholics Anonymous.

TJ had ten admissions for intentional drug overdoses and alcohol withdrawal within 12 months. He was first labeled a "hateful patient" when he was admitted to the hospital after telling his outpatient psychiatrist that he had eaten multiple boxes of rat poison with the intention of killing himself. Many more admissions due to sequelae of rat poison ingestion would follow. TJ wanted to be on the psychiatric unit, not the general medical floor, but previous psychiatric admissions were not therapeutic; that is, admission to a short-term psychiatry unit only provided temporary relief for problems that were still present once TJ was discharged. During

---

* Ted Jacobs is not the patient's real name; it was changed to protect the patient's privacy.

a lengthy admission to stabilize him hematologically, TJ wreaked havoc among the medical teams, especially medicine and C-L psychiatry.

The patient frustrated the medicine team when only intravenous, not oral, vitamin K would bring his prothrombin time closer to normal limits. When it became clear that TJ was not swallowing his oral medication but was destroying it after the nurse left (although he denied it), frustration turned to anger, fueled further by TJ's refusal to go voluntarily to the county crisis stabilization facility (CSF) where all county mental health patients are sent when they are involuntarily assessed for transfer to an inpatient psychiatric unit in the county, for discharge, or for short-term stabilization. As long as TJ needed an IV, he could not go to the CSF. Despite the anger and turmoil that surrounded him and that in part was generated by him, TJ talked about the hospital as "a safe environment" versus his apartment, which he described as "a black hole I crawl into at night and can't come out of until morning."

The medicine team was extremely frustrated with the patient and with the psychiatry team, which did not "fix" the patient, did not accept him on the psychiatry unit, and did not get him permanently discharged. C-L psychiatry, recognizing the "splitting behavior" that is part of BPD, was frustrated by TJ's behaviors and the medicine service. (Splitting behavior is a coping process in which an individual pits one entity against another.) Medical students on the internal medicine rotation were so overwhelmed by the patient's behavior and the resulting discord that they presented him to the weekly internal medicine ethics conference twice with the C-L psychiatrist present. Many staff had talked with the clinical ethicist (JDS) about TJ, and a formal ethics consult was requested to help the medicine service focus on what was best for the patient – that is, respect him as an individual and help him make "safe" decisions for himself.

The ethicist worked with C-L psychiatry to help mediate the consequences of the splitting behaviors, which were unacceptably recorded in TJ's chart. The behaviors were harmful not only to TJ but also to relationships between staff and potentially to the institution legally. Following are examples of the frustration displayed in TJ's chart by a member of the medicine team: "I am still not clear how psychiatry evaluates a patient for suicidal potential, as every time they say it is OK to send patient home, patient comes back in not more than three days. Is there any way to predict at least one week?" and, "His mood is much improved, believe it or not, since admission." The potentially harmful notes in TJ's record were discontinued when the real and potentially negative outcomes of the comments were made clear to all involved.

Members of the staff realized that the dynamics of their interactions with this patient were different from other patients and that relationships among staff were increasingly strained. Fortunately, the relationship between the psychiatry attending and internal medicine (IM) was not as strained as it could have been because the IM attending was a personal friend of KSW (and JDS). However, this relationship increased the pressure to manage TJ's care effectively and to provide relief for the IM service in dealing with this difficult patient.

Despite the anger and frustration brought about by TJ's behaviors, empathy was rekindled when TJ talked about his loneliness and how his father never paid attention to him. TJ wondered aloud what it would take to get his father to show he cared. KSW wondered if he would find out before he died. The psychiatrist and ethicist worked with staff members to help them understand how sick and lonely TJ was and how badly he needed our care, but with carefully set, and consistently maintained, boundaries.

Respecting his right to make decisions for himself was difficult because we could not know when to believe that he would not harm himself. When discussing discharge planning, TJ made it clear he did not want to leave the hospital. He refused a group home and refused to sign himself into the CSF voluntarily. At the time of discharge, he continued to refuse available options and was sent involuntarily to the CSF. He returned to the hospital five days later due to nosebleeds (from the rat poison) and told us that the CSF had released him 45 minutes after he arrived. This admission became even more serious when it was discovered TJ had ingested cadmium (while denying he had eaten batteries). TJ manipulated the system, not seeming to care whether he lived or died. He appeared to be almost euphoric to be in the hospital despite complaints of boredom.

The ethicist and the C-L psychiatrist worked with staff individually and in groups to facilitate a healthy ventilation of their anger – especially after a nurse yelled at the C-L psychiatrist about getting TJ, who smoked, off suicide precautions. This would cut down on her work because patients on suicide precautions must be assessed every 15 minutes and must be accompanied by staff to smoke outside. We made Groves' article, "Taking Care of the Hateful Patient," available to staff and worked to identify the negative and positive aspects of labeling.[1] We also asked staff members what they believed they could do to help this man while recognizing that patients with a BPD diagnosis have been labeled "the hemophiliacs of emotion" in the literature due to the extraordinary amount of time and energy they consume.[2]

It was clear TJ harmed himself more dramatically each time he was discharged from the hospital, and we did our best to help TJ, but anything we did was undermined by the patient. The needs of staff and of the patient collided; staff members felt they were going in circles. Groves described how "a psychologically naïve medical staff may regress to a helpless or vengeful position in response to the patient's ingratitude, intractability, impulsivity, manipulativeness, entitlement and rage."[3] Groves' description was accurate in describing how those involved with Ted Jacob often felt.

TJ had more admissions to our institution before he was finally committed (to our collective relief) to the state psychiatric hospital by the CSF because of his escalating self-destructive behavior. TJ continued his destructive behavior at the state hospital. He placed a plastic bag over his head but was found before he was harmed. The entire ward was placed on suicide precautions as a consequence, which resulted in other patients on the unit being angry at TJ and the staff.

TJ was discharged and readmitted to medical and psychiatric units several more times both in and out of his hometown. Six months after TJ's last admission to our hospital, many of us involved in his care were sobered to read his starkly brief obituary in the local newspaper.

Ted Jacob, age 39 years, died suddenly in [large Midwestern city] where he had resided the last 6 months. He was employed as a carpenter and previously as a construction worker. He is survived by his father, wife, and brother. He was preceded in death by his mother. There will be no visitation and interment will be private.[4]

Professional reflections

The authors were not immune to strong feelings about both the patient and the staff. Our feelings covered a wide range, from impotence at not being able to protect the patient from himself – which we recognized was not always possible – to deep frustration with a system that was unable to protect TJ from harming himself. We were both amazed at the patient's tenacity. For example, he took massive doses of warfarin when he swallowed the rat traps, he overdosed on chlorpromazine (an antipsychotic), he swallowed batteries, and drank heavily. We did not try to guess what he might do next, as he was both creative and tenacious.

We were also frustrated with the notes written by the internal medicine residents in the patient's record. This was particularly disturbing for KSW, as the notes became increasingly more inappropriate and personal toward psychiatry than toward the ethics consultant.

JDS was frustrated at the unprofessional and unethical behavior of many of the staff, including physicians who were involved with the patient's care. Unfortunately, staff was noisily angry at each other in open areas of the nursing station, where comments could be overheard by other patients and families. While we recognized the staff was ventilating its frustration and anger, this was not the appropriate place to do it, which had been discussed on numerous occasions. When health professionals need to express anger, a private room is better than an area where angry words can be overheard, potentially harming both the staff and the patient. There were also times when JDS became caught up in the splitting behaviors and had to step back to regain some balance. While both the psychiatrist and ethicist were glad to see progress in the recognition of splitting behaviors, this progress could vanish quickly when TJ flaunted his destructive behaviors. The phrase "hateful patient" blossomed for JDS in working with TJ and the staff. Working closely with the psychiatrist was helpful and supportive. Working with the staff was difficult and frustrating, but it was also productive and fruitful.

Another issue was the hospital "grapevine," which raised serious ethical issues about how negative labels are used and the harm they may cause. Fortunately, in this situation, the article we distributed by Groves facilitated discussion of the label of "hateful patient" and helped increase the staff's awareness of the dynamics of TJ's situation. It was evident that most of the health professionals who worked with TJ felt anger and frustration. Increasing staff's awareness of how feelings were expressed and how to deal with them – even on a small scale – seemed to be helpful.

After reading about TJ's death in the starkly grim obituary, we stepped back from the chaos he had generated and agreed that we learned important lessons from him about caring for very difficult patients. He helped us acknowledge that there are times when we will feel powerless because we cannot protect patients from their self-destructive behaviors. TJ reinforced our belief in the importance of thoughtful early intervention with healthcare professionals and patients to pre-empt the splitting behaviors seen in patients with BPD, which can irrevocably distort relationships between patients and staff and among healthcare profession-als. While TJ forced us to identify biases and limitations (as mentioned throughout this article) that affect how we care for such challenging patients, TJ also left us with the nagging question of whether there was anything more, any other intervention, that we could have implemented to save him.

Haunting aspects

TJ clearly left us, and some of the staff, wondering what – if anything – we might have done to help him, to prevent what we suspect was a sad and lonely time leading to a grim and lonely death. We saw signs of his loneliness on virtually each admission to our hospital. KSW had commented in an early admission that TJ would die before he got positive attention from his adopted father, but we were not able to help him reach his emotionally distant father. We also could understand why his father would choose to distance himself from TJ. TJ was difficult for us to deal with as a team, and his father was trying to live his own life without the life-threatening behaviors of the son he had agreed to adopt years before.

TJ's desperate acts to stay in the hospital, a "safe," more caring environment, intermittently haunt us. It is accepted that patients who are frequently in the hospital may view certain staff as family members and the hospital as a home. TJ was desperate to stay in the hospital, which he said was more like a home to him than the apartment he described as "a black hole." When we could step back from our frustration and impatience with his behaviors, TJ was like a hauntingly sad child without a true home or anyone to love him or care about him. When I (JDS) am consulted today to deal with problems arising from the desperate behaviors of a patient with BPD, I think of TJ, and I talk about the seriousness of behavior using TJ's story as an example of a haunting outcome.

Outcome

The most obvious outcome of this case was TJ's death. His obituary had a significant effect on many of us – largely because of its starkness and how it exemplified his life for his caregivers.

As noted earlier, we (JDS and KSW) learned many lessons from TJ – as did the staff and other physicians involved in caring for him. The primary internal medicine attending still uses TJ as an example in his teaching on rounds – especially the ethical issues that can arise from what is written in a patient's chart and how patients deserve our care even when difficult or "hateful." The importance of setting boundaries is frequently addressed on rounds when JDS is present. TJ has certainly left us with the nagging reality that our healthcare system is not designed to save everyone, especially when patients are ambivalent about whether they want to live or receive care. This raises the final issue of how much responsibility and how many resources healthcare professionals should invest in protecting such patients? In the end, it did not appear there were enough resources available to adequately protect TJ.

Discussion questions

1. What processes or techniques can a clinical ethics consultant or committee use with angry, frustrated staff members who are dealing with exceptionally difficult or "hateful" patients?
2. What are the most common ethical problems likely to arise with difficult patients?
3. What – or who – are useful resources for working with difficult patients?
4. How would you recommend that a clinical ethics consultant deal with feelings generated by working with patients labeled as difficult?
5. How would you balance the ethical principles mentioned at the beginning of this paper (i.e., respect for persons and autonomy, nonmaleficence, and beneficence) in this case?

REFERENCES

1. Groves JE. Taking care of the hateful patient. *N Engl J Med*, 1978; 298: 883–7.
2. Straus H. Hemophiliacs of emotion. *Am Health*, 1998; 7: 61–6.
3. Groves JE. Difficult patients. In: Cassem NH, Stern TA, Rosenbaum JF, Jellinek MS, eds. *Massachusetts General Hospital Handbook of General Hospital Psychiatry*, 4th ed. Chicago: Mosby Year Book, 1997; 337–66.
4. The obituary was edited to preserve the patient's family's privacy.

10

Ulysses contract

Barbara J. Daly and Cynthia Griggins

Case narrative

Jimmy was a 24-year-old man who experienced a spinal cord injury at C-3 from a gunshot wound during a drug deal two years ago, resulting in quadriplegia. Following the initial acute-care episode and a stay in a rehabilitation facility he was transferred to a nursing home for long-term care. He was cognitively intact, ventilator dependent, and had developed multiple pressure ulcers (sacrum, heel, calf). He had a diverting colostomy and suprapubic bladder catheter. He had had a percutaneous gastrotomy (PEG) tube inserted during the initial acute hospitalization. Although he was able to eat, tube feedings were used as needed to supplement his oral intake and to assure adequate nutrition. He was able to exhale sufficient air around his tracheostomy to whisper short sentences.

Jimmy had no siblings. His mother lived in another city and visited infrequently. He had several friends who remained in contact with him for the first year after his injury but who no longer visited or called.

Jimmy intermittently refused to allow dressings on his pressure ulcers to be changed. The prescribed routine included daily dressing changes to the deep sacral wound and every other day changes of moisture-barrier dressings on his heel and calf ulcers. The sacral pressure ulcer covered the entire area of one buttock and extended part of the way across the top of the other buttock. It was a stage 4 wound, with persistent infection. A foul odor was evident in his room when Jimmy refused to allow wound care. Jimmy had to be turned completely on his side to provide access to the wound so the dressing could be changed. This required packing with sterile dressings and covering. Although he had no feeling in the wound itself, Jimmy complained that he felt like he could not breathe when he was turned on his side for the dressing changes.

Jimmy had several episodes of sepsis, thought to be related to infection of his wounds, prior to his hospitalization with us. These blood infections were life-threatening, though they had been successfully treated with antibiotics each time. The nursing home staff attempted multiple strategies to help Jimmy tolerate the dressing changes, including making various changes to his ventilator settings and even giving him intravenous medication for "conscious sedation" during dressing changes. Despite these efforts, he continued to refuse turning and dressing changes for days at a time, sometimes as long as a week. He eventually developed pneumonia and became hemodynamically unstable. Because he steadfastly insisted that he wanted to live and refused to agree to a do-not-attempt-resuscitation (DNAR) order, he was transferred to the intensive-care unit (ICU) at our hospital. His pneumonia and sepsis were treated and his condition stabilized, but he continued to refuse to be turned or to have his dressings changed. An ethics consultation was requested by the ICU team.

A conversation was held with Jimmy about his reasons for refusing and his goals for treatment. He insisted that he wanted to "get better" and go back to the nursing home, but he "couldn't stand" the dressing change because of how it made him feel. He continued to refuse a DNAR order. After we repeated this conversation several times over the next few days and after we attempted several techniques to assure that Jimmy's ventilation was not compromised by turning, Jimmy was asked to choose his most important goal of treatment: prolonged survival or avoiding the discomfort of dressing changes. He again chose survival.

At this point the ethics consultant explained that the only way we could promote his goal (survival) was to provide adequate wound care, including turning for regular dressing changes. Therefore, if he wanted us to support this goal, we would institute a "Ulysses contract," specifying the plan to change his dressings once a day. Each day he could request the time at which the dressings were changed, but we would not honor a refusal. The contract would be renegotiated once a week. At this time he could change his mind about his goals or renegotiate the exact terms. We also included some aspects of care in the contract that were important to him, such as control over some of his medications, the choice of special foods he liked, having a fan in his room, and assigning the nurses he preferred. Agreeing to a contract was the only way we would be willing to continue his care in the ICU. If he did not agree to the contract, we would discharge him to the nursing home because continued care in the ICU would serve no purpose. We also explicitly discussed the options of hospice or palliative care and assured him of adequate comfort measures if he ever changed his mind about his goals. He indicated that he understood and repeated his wish to survive.

The contract was agreed upon, and for the first few days Jimmy accepted the dressing changes, and the promises of the staff regarding his care were fulfilled. On the fourth day after initiating the contract, Jimmy objected to the dressing change. His objection was overridden, as outlined in the contract, he was positioned on his side, and his dressings were changed. At the end of seven days, the contract was renewed.

Professional reflections

This case presented a number of challenging issues that occur with some frequency: how to assist patients who pass formal competency evaluations yet seem unable to process information and to choose rationally; how to balance the competing demands of autonomy and beneficence; how to balance the rights of one patient against the rights of others; and how to determine the limits of professional responsibility to patients who refuse medically necessary care. What made Jimmy's case unique was the combination of all of these elements coupled with his profound vulnerability and life-threatening illness. Given his quadriplegia and lack of family advocates, he was truly at the mercy of healthcare professionals and his life was in the balance.

Jimmy had been consistently evaluated by psychiatrists and determined to have adequate capacity to make his own medical decisions. He demonstrated a reasonably good understanding of his condition, the risks of infection, and the necessity of treating his wounds. Jimmy clearly expressed his desire to live, although he was not able to articulate his values and reasoning in any detail. He seemed to understand the consequences of his decisions. And yet when faced with an uncomfortable procedure he seemed equally unable to appreciate how his refusal of care at that moment would prevent realization of what he identified as his most important goal – to survive.

As we worked to understand this paradox, it occurred to us that Jimmy's situation seemed analogous to Ulysses. In moments of calm rationality, he was clear about wanting to act prudentially. Yet when his rational abilities were overwhelmed by external forces (in his case, the discomfort and perhaps fear engendered by the dressing changes), he was unable to adhere to his earlier commitment. Thus, the idea of offering a "Ulysses contract" to Jimmy was born. Ulysses contracts are a form of precommitment enacted by a person, typically with intermittent psychosis. The contracts detail plans to disregard requests issued during the period of irrationality.[1] As in the original Greek tale of Ulysses, these contracts are established between the person with the predictable impairment and a trusted ally, typically a physician with whom the patient has an established relationship. These agreements, sometimes called "psychiatric advance directives," have been used to authorize the professional to make decisions on such things as hospitalization, use of psychotropic medications, or other forms of treatment over the objections of the patient.[2]

Ulysses contracts have been the subject of debate in bioethics, law, and psychiatry. Proponents argue that such contracts are justified to protect patients from future impairment that poses serious threats to important interests, including physical safety and well-being. The contract can be an effective protection against mental incapacity. Opponents point out that the effect of enforcing a contract that overrides present wishes in favor of previous choices is an unjustified violation of autonomy and usually imposes the health professional's preference for the previous choice. Importantly, unlike advance directives used to indicate end-of-life choices, Ulysses contracts are enforced while the person still retains some decisional capacity. This is done so intervention can take place before the patient's condition has progressed to total incompetence and harm has resulted. Thus, Ulysses contracts are specifically intended to limit autonomous choices in ways that are usually prohibited by the principle of respect for autonomy and to protect the individual not only from mental impairment, but also from *akrasia*, or weakness of will.[3]

Contracting with patients to influence behavior is a common practice. Typically, contracts are a means of explicitly outlining expectations and boundaries for behavior, providing the patient with acceptable ways and areas in which he/she can exert some control over his/her care, and often (though not always) including some incentives for adhering to the terms of the contract. Contracts are intended to provide a means of respecting the patient's right to voluntarily enter into agreements regarding elements of medical care while also protecting the right of the institution and its staff to be free from abuse and to establish conditions needed for the provision of effective care.[4] Such contracts have no legal force and primarily function as a behavior-modification intervention, providing structure for both the patient and the professional staff. Unlike Ulysses contracts, they can be revoked at any time and are actually based on the assumption that the patient retains both the rights and responsibilities of a competent adult.

The use of a Ulysses contract with Jimmy stemmed first from our assessment that his wish to survive was sincere and deeply held. Jimmy was consistent in stating that he wanted to live, and he never wavered in his refusal of treatment limitations and hospice referral. Second, we believed that while Jimmy did not lack decisional capacity in the formal sense, his insight into his own behavior and motivations, as well as his inability to see beyond the moment or to tolerate brief current discomfort for the sake of future long-term goals, was significantly impaired. Third, we had a high degree of certainty that the dressing changes were essential if we were to prevent recurrent sepsis, which would eventually end his life. Finally, we believed that we were not obligated to deliver care that was significantly substandard.

Haunting aspects

Many aspects of Jimmy's story continue to haunt us. Some are related to Jimmy's nightmarish situation; others have to do with our response – the Ulysses contract – and our lingering doubts about whether we had respected or disrespected Jimmy in making such a contract.

Coming face to face with patients' vulnerability is always humbling. But facing the significant powerlessness of the quadriplegic, especially a previously healthy young man like Jimmy, fills us with discomfort. Most patients, even at their sickest, can still express their feelings, resist their fate, or protect themselves in some way – by yelling, cursing, or striking out. But ventilator-dependent quadriplegics can do none of these things. Indeed, Jimmy could only protest what was done to him by frowning, violently shaking his head, or grimacing. Jimmy had an extraordinary care team at the nursing home who respected refusals of care, but we were no longer doing this. Knowing that Jimmy was at our mercy, and seeing his discomfort and desperate pleas to be left alone (and to preserve his life) when we "enforced" the contract left us feeling a combination of guilt and disquietude. As clinicians, we (ethics consultants) were acting contrary to a deeply rooted norm – laying hands, so to speak, on a person against his expressed wishes. As ethicists, we were authorizing other staff, through our advice and recommendations, to do the same.

Making matters even worse was the fact that Jimmy had no one – no spouse, no relative, no close friend – looking after his welfare. Jimmy was truly alone in the world. This was not Christopher Reeve, who had an army of family, friends, physicians, and therapists helping him in his struggle to survive as a person with quadriplegia. Jimmy was much more typical of the population with quadriplegia: young, poor, and without the supports to build a meaningful life for himself in his paralysis. Where was justice? Would more socially connected patients have found themselves in this situation? Would the love and support of family and friends serve to motivate Jimmy or to protect him from the depths to which he had sunk? Would we have even entered into the Ulysses contract if a relative had been there protesting and supporting Jimmy when he refused to be turned?

As we reflect, we are also haunted by the questionable circumstances under which we "negotiated" the Ulysses contract with Jimmy. When he came to the hospital and faced more turning and dressing changes, what freedom did Jimmy really have to make medical decisions? We were clear: If he did not agree to the contract, he could not stay in the ICU and he would have to go back to his nursing home. Did this allow for *voluntary* choice? We were also concerned about Jimmy's level of understanding. He appeared to understand cognitively, but did he really grasp that his later refusal would be ignored? Did he realize that at least until the next negotiation he would not have a choice and would be turned no matter how he protested? In other words, did he know we were serious about this?

We were also uncomfortable because, to our knowledge, no one has negotiated a Ulysses contract with anyone but a psychiatric patient. We wondered if one could ethically do such a thing. Jimmy did not have a psychiatric disorder with waxing and waning mental capacity. He was not a competent person who became incompetent during a dressing change. He was simply an immature young adult who presumably had a very low tolerance for pain, anxiety, and discomfort. Therefore, on what basis were we entitled to ignore Jimmy's pleas to be left alone when it came time for dressing changes? Was the fact that he lacked the will or the fortitude to face the treatments sufficient? Does one have to be rendered "incompetent" by the pull of the sirens, or is their emotional power over a weak-willed person enough to justify being tied to the mast? As we pondered this question, we also asked ourselves whether labeling the agreement a "Ulysses contract" was an ethical ploy designed to get an immature and emotionally weak patient to do what we wanted and needed to do?

Our own motivation to negotiate a contract with Jimmy leaves us with some further questions. Healthcare professionals are committed to providing good care. In fact, they are ethically required to provide a certain standard of care. To do less not only violates professional codes of ethics, it also leaves the professional vulnerable to legal action. Therefore, when the nursing home and hospital staff requested an ethics consultation, in part it was to address their dilemma: Are they required to honor patient wishes if this means providing substandard care?

And what if that substandard care results in discomfort for other patients by causing unpleasant odors? The questions of other patients' comfort and the judicious use of resources are always difficult, but the amount of time and energy required to care for Jimmy aroused unusual levels of resentment and frustration among the healthcare team. Isolating a screaming or malodorous patient so other patients might not be disturbed is a common problem and it depends on available resources. In fact, the time and energy required to care for Jimmy was probably no more than a very complicated medical patient might require. The problem, of course, is that highly trained intensivists and critical-care nurses are not trained to handle behavioral problems. In their view, patients with behavioral difficulties are not as deserving of effort as medically complicated patients, nor are they as rewarding. Jimmy might have done better on a medical-behavioral unit, where such an expenditure of time and energy to deal with the complex interaction of physical and behavioral problems is more the norm.

Finally, we are haunted by the experience of carrying out a Ulysses contract. In the original tale, when Ulysses asked his crew to tie him to the mast, he instructed them to ignore his protests at the time of the Sirens' call. The crew's advantage over our modern-day healthcare professionals was that Ulysses' sailors all had wax in their ears to protect them from the Sirens' call. Therefore they could not hear Ulysses' pleas and protestations, which was probably a blessing. On the other hand, healthcare professionals who negotiate a Ulysses contract with a patient then must carry it out without the benefit of wax in their ears. They must witness and endure the patient's pleas, resistance, and anger when the contract must be enforced. The very nature of a Ulysses contract suggests that this is going to be unpleasant, a challenge to the healthcare professional used to honoring patient autonomy. We had no idea how difficult this would be. The support of the ethics committee and of our colleagues could not ameliorate the feelings aroused by holding down a protesting patient who felt like he might suffocate under our beneficence.

Outcome

The Ulysses contract remained in force for two-and-a-half weeks. At that time Jimmy called the ethics consultant back and stated that he wished to cancel the contract and change his goal to "comfort care" (i.e., DNAR order and a goal of maximizing comfort). After a long discussion in which Jimmy again refused to discuss his thinking in any detail, we agreed to his change. His anxiolytics were increased and he was allowed to refuse dressing changes. He was transferred to the nursing home with this plan in place. Once there, Jimmy changed his mind and asked that the DNAR be rescinded. This was done and he resumed refusing the dressing changes. When he became septic again in three weeks, he was transferred to a different hospital where he received all aggressive efforts to treat his sepsis. Despite this, he died after one week in the ICU.

Discussion questions

1. Were Jimmy's rights violated by the imposition of the Ulysses contract?
2. Were there other acceptable alternatives?
3. What might provide justification for not honoring his treatment refusal?
4. To what degree should an ethics consultant consider discomfort of other patients when giving ethics advice about one patient?

REFERENCES

1. Dresser R. Bound to treatment: The Ulysses contract. *Hastings Cent Rep*, 1984; 14(3): 13–16.
2. Srebnik DS, Rutherford LT, Peto T, *et al.* The content and clinical utility of psychiatric advance directives. *Psychiatr Serv*, 2005; 56: 592–8.
3. Spellecy R. Reviving Ulysses contracts. *Kennedy Inst Ethics J*, 2003; 13: 373–92.
4. Harris PS, Duermeyer M, Ehly C, *et al.* The "impossible patient": Organizational response to a clinical problem. *J Clin Ethics*, 1999; 10: 242–6.

11

Misjudging needs: a messy spiral of complexity

Paul J. Ford

Case narrative

Mr. William Winthorpe, a 60-year-old patient, was admitted to the hospital with ischemic brain injury secondary to an unwitnessed cardiopulmonary arrest.* He had a medical history of end-stage kidney, liver, and heart failure, needing chronic dialysis three times a week. In the first week at the intensive-care unit (ICU) after the arrest, a neurologist told Mr. Winthorpe's sons and daughters that, based on brain imaging, Mr. Winthorpe had no real chance of waking up or regaining any significant cognitive function. Although he was not brain dead, Mr. Winthorpe would have no significant cognitive recovery. The family was about to agree to withdraw aggressive therapies when the patient began to respond to external stimuli. These events occurred prior to my involvement as a clinical ethics consultant and set the context for the events that followed.

Several weeks after the arrest, and after the patient was discharged from the ICU to a regular hospital ward, a hospitalist requested a clinical ethics consultation. According to the hospitalist, the family did not understand the futility of current aggressive therapies. The hospitalist said Mr. Winthorpe sooner or later would die from an infection if not from his other end-stage organ diseases. At the time of the consultation the patient had begun to follow basic commands, which the family interpreted as the potential for meaningful recovery.

When I met with Mr. Winthorpe's family and medical team, the family expressed a desire to see how much cognition he could regain given that the original neurologist had been wrong about the impossibility of cognitive improvement. His family said, "If he improved some this week, then why can't he improve more? Now, if we knew he wouldn't get any better than he is, then of course we would stop. However, we gotta give him a fair shake. First, we need to see how much better he'll

---

* Many details have been omitted from this case in order to protect the confidentiality of the patient.

A version of this chapter was originally published in *The Journal of Clinical Ethics*, 16(3): 206–11.

get." After several discussions, there was agreement to allow more time (with no mention of duration) to evaluate whether the patient's cognition would improve. I entered several brief chart notes during my several days of involvement. My final note indicated that I was signing off the case. Subsequently, the patient moved between several different hospital units, with each new medical team having the same futile discussion with the family. After a number of weeks, the patient was discharged to an outside nursing facility after being able to say a few basic words and recognize family members. Since I had signed off and entered a clear chart note about the agreed-upon course, I was unaware of these events.

A month after the first ethics consult, the patient was readmitted to the hospital, but he was now no longer responsive. Another ethics consultation was called to facilitate a family meeting because an intensivist believed current therapy was futile. Since I was no longer "on service," the consult went to another ethics consultant. The ethics consultant reviewed the case, went to see Mr. Winthorpe, and spoke with the medical team. Our institution runs an individual ethics consultant model with a backup of a small group ethics committee review. Given that we strongly recommend that the small group ethics committee consult be used when an attending physician contemplates withdrawing therapies based on futility, the individual consultant recommended that this attending intensivist call a committee consult. Despite articulating that the current course of therapy was futile, the attending physician did not follow the recommendation to move the consultation to the committee level and continued aggressive therapy. Bioethics again signed off on the case given that the attending physician and the family were willing to continue current therapies. The patient subsequently was transferred to a regular nursing floor within the hospital.

A month after the second consult, another attending intensivist requested an ethics consultation. The patient's dialysis catheter had stopped functioning properly, and the intensivist believed that placing a new catheter constituted an inappropriate escalation of therapy. Given the patient's grim prognosis due to his multiorgan system failure and neurological devastation from the cardiac arrest, the intensivist judged reinstituting dialysis to be against standard medical practice.[1] The request for an ethics consultation prompted not only another individual ethics consultation (I was back on service) but also an ethics committee review for futility.

After another four weeks of discussion, debate, and posturing, the patient again started following basic commands (such as eye opening). Two weeks after this cognitive improvement, the patient was discharged again to a skilled nursing facility. Prior to this final discharge, it was decided by the medical staff, in consultation with bioethics, that since the patient would not benefit from further ICU intervention in the future he would not be readmitted to the ICU at our institution. The family agreed that the patient would not be returned to the hospital's ICU.

Haunting aspects

This case spanned several months. Many ethics questions arose and dissipated, persisted, or were resolved. Ethicists, physicians, ombudsmen, nurses, general counsel, and family members all attempted to resolve these issues. The case appears generic in many respects because it centers on the appropriate use of intensive medical treatments for a patient with multiorgan system failure in the presence of extensive ischemic brain injury. The invocation of futility in cases such as this one continues to be widely debated.[2,3,4,5] For me, futility of medical treatment is not the central haunting element. The interface between the family and the medical institution, as well as the nonlinear and unpredictable course of this terminal illness, were the most troubling aspects of the case. Although the outcome of the patient's illness was inevitable, the path to that inevitability was strewn with false indicators, missteps, and misunderstandings. The messy complexity resisted categorization of the case into a single ethics question.[6] From an ethics consultation process point of view this case raises questions about an ethicist's role, ethicists inserting themselves into situations, appropriate length of continued involvement, and what counts as a good outcome in ethics consultation. These process questions haunt me. Our system of ethical checks and balances may, in the end, have functioned as intended, but this case demonstrates elements needing improvement. A suboptimal outcome of this consultation should prompt a re-evaluation of the frequent lack of proactive efforts in clinical ethics consultation.[7]

The patient survived to discharge (twice) with some ability to cognitively "be in the world," that is, to react and respond with some level of intention. At base, this was good since the patient's life was extended and the family valued additional time spent with the patient. However, the case took several months and hundreds of hours of time from institutional employees and family members to resolve. Hospital security was called to address several disturbances surrounding pictures and recordings taken by the family. Several family members involved the ombudsman's office because of frustrations with the medical team. There were threats of court action and considerable negotiations. Although one family member was a legal decision-maker, documents in the chart listed another family member as the decision-maker. The confusion prompted anxiety and frustration in the family. These were all "bad" outcomes in terms of experiences of participants in the process. The anxiety, animosity, and stress negatively affected all involved parties. As I ponder the outcome, I do not feel pride that I helped navigate and resolve a particularly complex case. I feel dread, powerlessness, and frustration because of the excess negative emotions generated by so many individuals over such a long duration. In retrospect, there must have been better ways to resolve or at least more peacefully cope with the situation. Given the current reactive model of consultation this case could easily repeat itself, which haunts me. Although the process works well in most cases, it fails to be fully effective in some cases, even if an equitable, fair, and just end arises.

I empathized with the family's frustration that each new medical team asked the family to come to the hospital (during working hours) to have the same discussion about withdrawing therapies because of futility. Each new team believed that the family must not "understand" the situation. If they had, they certainly would withdraw all therapy. This was despite prior ethics consultation notes placed in the chart detailing the first ethics consultation with the family, including comments regarding the family's understanding. Although each team began to enact a plan of action agreed to by family and medical staff, the next medical team felt obligated to re-evaluate. Each medical team's desire for firsthand knowledge of the family's rationale placed a tremendous burden on the family.

Finally, this case haunts me from a policy viewpoint. I understand the family's desire to discover how much cognitive improvement the patient could attain before deciding on continuing aggressive therapies. When the patient's course did not follow what the original neurologist had predicted, the family began to doubt all medical judgments. According to the family, the patient was "stubborn." Because of this, the family interpreted the patient's periodic fluxes between minimal consciousness and unconsciousness as a desire to stay alive. The claim that a catheter occlusion moved the patient's treatments into the "futile" arena reinforced the family's skepticism and distrust. In spite of my understanding and empathizing with the family, I also understood the medical team's position that the patient's lifespan was extremely limited by his nonneurological illnesses and that they could do nothing but prolong dying. The ICU beds were full in that particular unit, and intensive-care physicians are trained to help patients overcome acute medical problems, not provide chronic intensive care. On these two points, the patient was considered medically inappropriate for continued ICU treatment by these doctors. Of course, this goes to the question of the purpose of ICUs in general and stewardship of resources. In an individual ethics case we usually avoid discussing resource allocation. However, too often this topic looms and is indirectly expressed. Until there is some consistency of policy applied to similar patients or there is a quantifiable shortage of ICU beds in an entire community, it would be inappropriate to appeal to futility to justify rationing in a particular case.

Professional reflections

The ethics consultation process was reactive rather than proactive. The first two consults were in the standard critical response mode that most ethics consultations take, that is, a value conflict had already occurred between parties, and the bioethicists were called upon to facilitate resolution of a problem. I wonder if a more careful and consistent follow-up of the original consultation would have resulted in a better situation. Perhaps I could have created a liaison that would have decreased animosity between the healthcare team(s) and the family. However, the clinical ethicist neither treats the patient nor is an "ethics cop" who interjects himself into a patient's case. In the end, uninvited interjection can be counterproductive to empowering physicians to address ethical challenges and can destroy trust with the medical team. Although collegially inquiring after a patient could avoid loss of trust, doing so may still encourage unneeded dependence. Even though the role and obligation of the ethics consultant changes once involved in a case, there are points at which the ethicist must trust professionals to enact plans that are put into place. In the current case, the ethics consultant had given guidance to the treating medical team during each consultation, but medical teams frequently rotate in large academic medical centers. The reactive nature of ethics consultation follows the model of many medical subspecialty consultations where the subspecialist consults on a single issue, gives recommendations within his/her sphere, and follows the case only to the extent the primary service requests. Given the limited time resources of ethics consultants, it is impractical to follow every ethics question and case until all value conflicts have been resolved. Consultation models are premised on the healthcare teams and patients being capable moral agents who only need assistance with subtle or complex issues.

The ethics consultation system is intended to facilitate resolution of complex value disagreements and to protect healthcare workers, patients, and families from unreflective decision making and abuses of power. However, attaining these goals can come at a significant emotional cost that should not be underestimated. With little way of knowing when the bioethics questions are fully answered for either chronic progressive or terminal illness, and with the need to rely on others to identify a need for ethics consultation cases, this type of case inevitably will arise again. I am skeptical that these important cases have good resolutions in the current model.

The idea that ethics consultations involve only small isolated questions within the dynamic hospital setting misunderstands the complex hospital environment. Except in published case write-ups, value/ethics issues are seldom well defined or limited to a single problem with a simple solution. The initial question consulted on in this case hinted at a variety of questions that arose throughout. In order to identify issues and dissect problems it was necessary to access a variety of information sources. Although being consulted on this case gave me a right to access the patient's medical information, I understood that access is limited to the amount necessary to discover all relevant ethics issues, to make recommendations, and to document those recommendations. My right of access required authorization, such as a request for a consult, from the medical team or patient. Being proactive in this case would have meant extending my access to patient records and activity, which was beyond the invitation extended by either the family or the medical team. Although in retrospect this might have facilitated a better process, it would have run the risk of overstepping professional boundaries with a continued assertion into the case beyond any identifiable ethics question. I was not asked to be a permanent advocate for this patient or to oversee medical treatment. To fall into the error of believing that an ethics consultant's role is only patient advocate is to forget the many other obligations to institutions, healthcare providers, and society. Further, I should not intrude on the privacy of a person's medical record simply for my own "closure." I take seriously my obligation to explore all of the relevant ethics questions in the case, articulate those problems, and give written recommendations and advice.

Outcome

Many months later, a family member contacted bioethics about a completely separate matter. The family member said the patient had died a couple of weeks after being discharged from our institution. The family had accepted this as a sad but expected outcome.

Currently as I sign off on complex cases, it is not uncommon for me to envision Mr. Winthorpe or one of his adult children. During those moments, I wonder if I am in the middle of another haunting case that will come back to the consultation service again and again. Retrospectively, it is simple to see lost opportunities to intervene in the process. As a consultant I continue to question whether, at each step in a complex case, there are ways to keep patients, families, and staff from spiraling into a messy complexity that will evade a good resolution and have high emotional cost. I am left with a knot in my stomach of not knowing.

Discussion questions

1. Should an ethics consultant ever follow a patient after the consultation episode is complete? Why or why not? If so, under what circumstances?
2. What should an ethics consultant do when his/her recommendations are not followed by the patient, medical team, or family?
3. Was there a possibility of a "good" ethics outcome in this case? How would this be measured (participant satisfaction, reduction in cost, minimized suffering)?
4. How extensively should the ethics consultant explore confidential medical records in order to get a full sense of the patient's progress? For instance, if there were a psychiatric note available in the case, what justification would be needed to review it?

REFERENCES

1. Moss A. (for the Renal Physicians Association and the American Society of Nephrology Working Group). Shared decision making in dialysis: A new clinical practice guideline to assist with dialysis-related ethics consultations. *J Clin Ethics*, 2001; 12(4): 406–14.

2. Council on Ethical and Judicial Affairs, American Medical Association. Guidelines for the appropriate use of do-not-resuscitate orders. *JAMA*, 1991; 265(14): 1868–71.
3. Cohen NH. Assessing futility of medical interventions – is it futile? *Crit Care Med*, 2003; 31(2): 646–8.
4. Hinshaw DB, Pawlik T, Mosenthal AC, Civetta JM, Hallenbeck J. When do we stop, and how do we do it? Medical futility and withdrawal of care. *J Am Coll Surg*, 2003; 196(4): 621–51.
5. Kurent JE. Case presentation: Medical decision-making in hopeless situations: The long-lost son. *J Pain Symptom Manage*, 2003; 25(2): 191–2.
6. Zaner RM. *Ethics and the Clinical Encounter*. Englewood Cliffs, NJ: Prentice Hall, 1988.
7. Miller RB. Extramural ethics consultation: Reflections on the mediation/medical advisory panel model and a further proposal. *J Clin Ethics*, 2002; 13(3): 203–15.

12

When the patient refuses to eat

Debra Craig and Gerald R. Winslow

The fundamental dynamics of this haunting case began long before the late-June day when the patient presented to our hospital for the first time. Perhaps they began when Mrs. Blue, at the age of 18, married a take-charge man she had known since her childhood. More recently, there was a significant day when Mr. Blue found the patient's mother wandering on foot in the slow lane of a busy freeway. Both of these details emerged as the story unfolded.

Case narrative

Mrs. Blue, 55 years of age, presented to our hospital on a summer day after her husband had arranged an appointment with our psychiatric outpatient clinic for eating disorders. The intake coordinator sent the patient to our emergency department after obtaining a history that the patient had not consumed any food and had taken in very little fluids during the last *ten* days.

Upon examination in the emergency room, Mrs. Blue was found to be volume depleted, with some renal insufficiency, electrolyte disorders, and hypoalbuminemia. She weighed 36.7 kg (81 lbs) and was 157 cm (5 ft) tall, resulting in a body-mass index (BMI) of 14.7. In other words, the patient weighed less than 67% of her expected body weight, indicating severe malnutrition. As a rule, when a person is approximately 60% of expected weight, death occurs. The team from internal medicine noted that she was alert, oriented, and in no apparent distress.

In late October of the previous year, this patient developed moderately severe headaches and visited her physician. Her husband reported that she had never had any serious illnesses. Breast augmentation surgery was the only surgical procedure she had undergone. She was up to date on recommended screening tests, she exercised regularly, and she consumed a consistently healthful diet. The patient took one dose of Motrin, 600 mg prescribed by the physician, and she noticed "burning in her stomach and sinuses." The next morning she called the doctor to report these symptoms. She took three more doses of the medication and then stopped due to the fact that "she had terrible abdominal pain and something was wrong with her GI tract and sinuses." From that time until she was seen in our hospital, she had neither eaten normally nor taken in fluids in keeping with her previous habits. Between late October and when we saw her in June, she had undergone complete evaluations in three different hospitals. She had also seen numerous physicians and had been treated for dehydration at several emergency rooms. Despite batteries of tests and procedures, no abnormalities were discovered. On one occasion, after presenting to another emergency room at a major academic facility, a psychiatrist was called. Mrs. Blue left against medical advice after her husband rejected the inpatient psychiatric facility the psychiatrist recommended.

Mr. Blue had taken much time away from his private business, and the patient's children, married and in their mid-20s, had "placed their lives on hold" while assisting with their mother's activities of daily living. Mr. Blue worked and maintained the home.

The day after Mrs. Blue's admission, a second-year psychiatry resident evaluated her carefully. She told the resident she could not eat because something was wrong with her stomach. His conclusions were Axis 1 – Psychosis versus psychotic depression versus anorexia nervosa. His recommendation, in addition to encouraging oral intake, was to offer the antipsychotic medication quetiapine for disorganized thoughts. The attending psychiatrist agreed with his plan via phone. However, the attending psychiatrist did not see the patient until almost five days later.

In my role as clinical ethicist, I (DC) was asked to see the patient four days after admission and three days after the psychiatric consult. I always require the requesting individuals to articulate the ethical dilemma and state what they would like me to address. This team replied, "Does she have decision-making capacity?" Behind this question was the obvious conflict between doing what was best for the patient from a medical perspective and respecting her right to refuse medical care if she had decision-making capacity.

I spoke with the patient at length at mid-afternoon on a Saturday. She was alone at the time. In fact, her family had been asked by the attending physician to refrain from visiting for 48 hours. His request reflected his opinion that an abnormal family dynamic focused on food and fluid might be adding to the patient's unwillingness to eat. When I met Mrs. Blue, she was seated in bed and dressed in a hospital gown. She was rail thin, pale, and she had an expressionless face. She seldom made or maintained eye contact. She spoke in a soft monotone. She had a tray of liquids, Jell-Os, puddings, and dietary supplements. Several containers were open three hours after mealtime, but none showed any sign of being consumed.

Mrs. Blue gave me the same history she had given others. She could not articulate her understanding of the risks of not eating or drinking. Her response to questions about risk was "I am working on it." Each time she would repeat the words "working on it" she would pick up one of the drinks, swirl it repeatedly, bring the straw to within millimeters of her lips, but not take a drink. She would put the drink down and look at me in a way that suggested she wanted praise or approval. Not once did the straw touch her lips. She consumed nothing during my 90-minute visit. She did not use the word "die" or acknowledge that not eating or drinking could lead to serious illness or death. She seemed entirely unable to look into the future. When I firmly pressed her about the future, she finally said she would like to spend time with her children and grandchildren. When I asked her if she would be willing to eat, drink, receive artificial feedings, or take medicine to accomplish this goal, she replied, "I would rather not." I was convinced that she was not able to understand, on a general or personal level, the risks of her behaviors or the consequences of her decisions. Therefore, she could not reason about treatment choices. In my estimation, she lacked decision-making capacity.

Before the interview ended, I tried to evoke a little emotion by asking her about the changes that had occurred in the lives of her husband and adult children as the result of her illness. Since she seemed largely unconcerned about herself, perhaps she would show concern for her loved ones. She denied any anxiety about them, saying only that her family was very supportive and gladly did what it could to help her.

When I was ready to end the session, I told Mrs. Blue that I did not believe she was making decisions in her best interest. I also told her I was going to indicate that I did not believe she had decision-making capacity, and I would recommend that someone else make decisions for her until she was well enough to make them for herself. It was only then that I felt even one moment of personal connection. She looked at me directly and asked me why I was making that recommendation. I said it was based on the conversation we just had. She smiled just a bit and then said, "If you're not pleased with our conversation then let's talk some more." I assured her I would be back to talk more with her.

I asked the patient's attending physician, an internist, on the day of my original consult to consider the diagnosis of psychotic depression and to bring up the topic of electroconvulsive therapy (ECT) with the psychiatry consultant and the patient's family. He suggested Mrs. Blue explore the option of ECT, but she refused. The attending physician agreed that the patient did not have adequate decision-making capacity.

I spoke to the patient's husband the next day. To be more accurate, I should say I listened to the husband for almost two hours. He was sad at the thought of losing his wife and was eager to find help for her. He was worried about the effect of her illness on the family and expressed his desire to have her well. He told me the story of a woman he had known since she was a child. She became the "perfect wife," the "perfect mother," and the "perfect hostess." Some time later she became the "perfect caregiver" for her demented mother. He was quick to tell me she wanted for nothing. He anticipated and supplied her every need. This left her free to concentrate on her beauty, her body, her hair, her diet, and her exercise program.

Another part of his long story gripped me. He told of driving along a busy freeway one day when he passed a car that appeared to be stalled. Traffic soon slowed to pass a person walking much too close to the lanes of traffic. It was his 55-year-old mother-in-law. She seemed confused but was able to tell him her car had stalled. When they returned to the car it was fully functional, running, and locked. She developed rapidly progressive dementia, was bedridden and mute within three years, and was maintained on artificial feeding for years. When I asked if Mrs. Blue was experiencing any signs or symptoms of forgetfulness, his response was a firm "No." He was quick to add that his wife had said many times that she did not want to end up like her mother.

Mr. Blue was conflicted. He felt like he had "spoiled" his wife. He felt it was his responsibility to make good decisions for her, but he did not want to override her decision and consent to force-feeding. Mr. Blue hired an attorney and filed for conservatorship, or what is commonly called guardianship. He also indicated that he would allow nasogastric (N-G) tube feeding beginning that day. However, Mr. Blue changed his mind almost immediately when the physicians arrived at the bedside and his wife remained adamant that she did not want the tube.

The next *four* days passed. Mrs. Blue still would not eat but would take occasional sips of liquid. She was receiving IV fluids, but she did not take any medicine. She continued to complain of worsening abdominal symptoms that were made worse after *any* oral intake. The attending psychiatrist, who had only heard of this patient through his resident, wrote a note in the chart, but he did not mention decision-making capacity. He commented that the patient denied being depressed and that she exhibited disorganized thinking with delayed thought processes. He recommended antipsychotic and antidepressant medications.

On the tenth day of hospitalization, Mr. Blue asked that his wife be discharged and stated that the accompanying nurse would be present in the home to supervise oral intake and care for the patient. On that day, the internal medicine team asked for a final decision about placement of an N-G tube. Mr. Blue again gave his permission to override his wife's objections and place the N-G tube. Right after this, the patient took in 400 cc of fluid before her husband changed his mind and withdrew permission for the N-G tube. After much discussion, the patient was finally discharged to home. She died nine days later.

Haunting aspects

This case is haunting for a number of reasons. First, we may have been obligated to delve deeper into various medical and motivational questions. Did Mrs. Blue die of an undiagnosed, untreated mental or physical disease? Was the patient in a state of psychotic depression? Was this a rare medical illness and could it have been treated? Was she for the first time in her life taking charge? Was this her way to exit life prior to suffering the indignities she witnessed in her mother's cognitive deterioration? These all involve uncertainties.

Most of the professional caregivers felt that Mrs. Blue did not have decision-making capacity, and they agreed that her husband was the "logical" decision-maker. Despite this, most caregivers were uncomfortable with the way her husband exercised his role. The team of caregivers was uncertain about how to interpret the actions of an individual who claimed such perfect love for his wife yet could not go against her wishes to save her life.

Without dismissing the valuable role of the physician trainee, resolution of a case as complex as Mrs. Blue's is best achieved through early and continued communication among various members of the attending physician staff. As I review this case, I am certain that I could have facilitated this communication by seeking a clearer statement from psychiatry on the patient's decision-making capacity and by urging psychiatry to act more definitively. In addition, asking legal counsel for a recommendation about seeking legal permission to provide nutrition may have prevented some of the distress caused to all parties by the vacillations of the patient's husband. I have wondered whether we erred in asking Mr. Blue to make a decision we felt was relatively simple but which, in his situation, he was incapable of making. Did we waste time waiting for an answer from Mr. Blue about feeding when Mrs. Blue's symptoms were probably that of a disease best treated by therapy (ECT) he could not consent to anyway (because surrogates may not consent to ECT on behalf of incompetent patients in our state)? Perhaps pursuing different guardianship than Mr. Blue through the court system would have resulted in ECT being performed.

Professional reflections

This case has triggered much reflection and discussion, in particular on the role of the ethics consultant. It may seem unusual for the ethics consultant to recommend a medical/psychiatric diagnosis and to suggest treatment as part of an ethics consult. Few of us wear only one hat. I (DC) am trained as an internist and geriatrician. I cannot ignore more than 20 years of practice. While some may argue that offering a recommendation about diagnosis and potential therapies goes well beyond the realm of answering the question about decision-making capacity, they are not easily separated. Establishing appropriate boundaries is complex. Consultants are invited guests whose recommendations do not have to be taken.

When, if ever, should we override a surrogate's decision-making authority? We are often confronted with patients whose chosen surrogates are no longer able to function effectively in that role. Often such cases involve elderly patients who have named a spouse or other family member as their agent. Over time, the agent becomes incapable of functioning as an effective surrogate. This may require seeking another agent than the one named on the patient's advance directive.

Clinical ethics would profit from a better understanding of why, when, and how to challenge the patient's surrogate.

Mrs. Blue's case illustrates our reluctance to override the decisions of adults who choose to end their lives by refusing to eat. This case also highlights the difficulty in dealing with patients whose physical difficulties are intertwined with psychological problems. It is often unclear how these interact and whether treating the psychological maladies against the will of the patient will ensure improvement. Mrs. Blue believed any oral intake caused unacceptable abdominal pain. We may think this is not so, or that it is psychosomatic, but patients are the final judge of whether they are experiencing pain. Mrs. Blue's case occurred in a legal jurisdiction that is influenced significantly by the case of Elizabeth Bouvia that unfolded about 20 years earlier.[1] In that case, the appellate court ruled that the patient had the legal right to refuse medically indicated nutrition and hydration even if not terminally ill. In the Bouvia case, the appellate court decided that her decision was not unreasonable given the poor quality of her life. With Mrs. Blue, it was difficult for observers to detect why her quality of life would be so unacceptable that she would starve herself to death. Of course, one could also wonder if it makes sense to talk about the patient "choosing" starvation if she lacks insight into the ramifications of her decisions. Perhaps the most salient lesson from this sad case is that there are limitations to what we can do to alter the poor decisions of our patients and their recognized surrogates.

Outcome

This case was reviewed in a monthly ethics committee meeting. The meeting occurred the day after Mrs. Blue's discharge. Several members of the committee feared she would soon die. Still, there was no agreement on a plan that could have prevented certain death.

Mrs. Blue left the hospital with her husband and a family friend who was also a private nurse. The day after discharge a physician referred them to a local hospice. The patient received hospice care, which was unusual given that she had no diagnosis of a terminal illness. The patient died at home nine days after discharge.

Mr. Blue expressed his sadness over the loss of his wife at a recent clinic visit. He said that he felt if his wife had received psychiatric care early in the course of her disease there may have been a different outcome. He said that he was at peace with the decision he and his children made not to force-feed Mrs. Blue.

Questions

1. Were Mr. Blue's vacillating decisions about the feeding tube an indication to challenge his capacity to serve as a surrogate decision-maker?

2. When is it the role of an ethics consultant to recommend medical treatment options?
3. What should trigger an ethics consultant to consult the hospital's legal counsel? Can doing so compromise the ethics consultation? Why or why not?

REFERENCE

1. *Bouvia v Superior Court (Glenchur)*, 179 Cal. App. 3d 1127, 225 Cal. Rptr. 297 (Ct. App. 1986), review denied (Cal. June 5, 1986).

Part IV

Withholding therapy with a twist

13

Listening to the husband

Ellen W. Bernal

Case narrative

An ethics consultation request with haunting features occurred at a Catholic hospital where I was on staff. I had collaborated with the chair of the medical-moral committee (as it was known at the time) and the hospital attorney (to whom I reported) to write my job description. My responsibilities included teaching, policy development, and availability for ethics consultations "in a manner similar to other medical consultations." Whether consultations would be carried out by an individual consultant, a small group, or the full ethics committee was to be decided. But before my arrival the small number of ethics consultations had been heard by the entire committee.

The first ethics consultation request came about two months after I was hired. Sr. Adrienne, director of pastoral care, related that a Catholic priest on staff was concerned about Ms. Barnes, a middle-aged woman with advanced chronic obstructive pulmonary disease (COPD) who was asking to be taken off ventilator support. The priest, Fr. Kelly, wanted to know: "How should we respond to requests to die in a Catholic hospital?" Sr. Adrienne was pleased to refer the question to me.

Several factors contributed to my discomfort with the ethics consult. I was new to the organization, and the position itself was new. Although I had years of teaching experience with healthcare professionals in a hospital setting, I had not been involved in ethics consultation itself. Given all this I felt a great sense of responsibility. I wanted to proceed cautiously and desired to attend to all details.

I recognized that ongoing contact with and guidance from the chair of the medical-moral committee and the hospital attorney were key. I asked both to confirm the consultation process: Obtain the attending physician's consent, identify the questions being asked, gather information, speak to all involved, convene a consultation meeting, and make a note in the chart with results. They also agreed to my request to speak about the case with an ethicist outside the institution. My plan was to provide background information for a full ethics committee review as had been done in the past.

Three days after Sr. Adrienne's call, Fr. Kelly and I spoke with Ms. Czerny, the nurse manager of the unit where Ms. Barnes was receiving care. Ms. Czerny confirmed that the patient had expressed a wish to stop ventilator support and recently was refusing blood draws and most food. Ms. Czerny related that Ms. Barnes was married and her husband was strongly opposed to her request to stop the ventilator. Ms. Czerny agreed that there was an ethical issue – namely the doctors' refusal to follow Ms. Barnes' request. She believed that Ms. Barnes was being treated against her will because the doctors feared a lawsuit.

Having determined that there was an ethical dilemma, as a courtesy I wanted to obtain permission from the attending physician to do an ethics consultation, even though the hospital chief executive officer (CEO) directed me to make ethics consultation services available to anyone directly involved with the care of a patient. "Would Ms. Czerny please ask Dr. Evans whether he would agree to the consultation, and if so, would he write a note to that effect in the patient's chart? When that is done, would Ms. Czerny please call legal services to verify that there was an appropriate record in the chart?" While this was going on, I spoke with the other ethicist about the case. The questions he identified were whether Ms. Barnes was able to make her own decisions and whether she understood the consequences. He recommended asking yes and no questions about the key issues and having a witness during the conversation. Ms. Czerny then related that Dr. Evans and Ms. Barnes had both agreed to the ethics consult, the chart note was in place, and Ms. Barnes still wanted to be taken off the ventilator. Legal services was trying to set up a meeting of several medical-moral committee members, which was surprisingly difficult. The medical-moral committee chair agreed that I could use an "individual consultant" model and call on others on an as-needed basis. Three days had now passed since Sr. Adrienne's original call.

I spoke with Dr. Evans the following day. He described Ms. Barnes as a "pulmonary cripple" who had been in and out of the hospital and on ventilator support for months. For the past six weeks and as recently as two days ago, she had expressed a wish to be taken off the ventilator. She did seem to understand that death would be the likely result. She did not write but could communicate by mouthing words. A recent psychiatric consult indicated she had decisional capacity. Dr. Evans said the family had initially been receptive to discontinuing life support, but now her husband was strongly opposed. At the same time, Mr. Barnes was not in favor of "full-code" status. Dr. Evans explained that it was not uncommon for him to withdraw ventilator support in end-stage COPD situations, but not when there is disagreement in the family. There was another problem. Ms. Barnes' ventilator dependence and her out-of-state medical insurance made it difficult to find an extended-care facility. Dr. Evans did not feel the need to meet with me and the patient but would be willing to participate in a medical-moral committee conference. He thought the committee might help facilitate family decision making, but he did not want us to make a recommendation.

The weekend elapsed. I hoped that efforts to "wean" the patient from the ventilator would succeed, causing the ethics consultation to "go away." However, on Monday nurses reported that during the ventilator weaning Ms. Barnes became very anxious and indicated that she wanted the machine set back to the usual rate. That same day I prepared to speak with Ms. Barnes. Her nurse said Ms. Barnes could mouth words and speak a little by blocking the tracheostomy for short periods. The nurse could usually understand her. I felt awkward. I had never tried to communicate with someone on a ventilator. Would I understand her? Was I asking the right questions? I was anxious about the seriousness of the decisions being made and worried about making a mistake.

Ms. Barnes was alert and in a chair when we entered her room. I asked yes and no questions and repeated her answers to be sure I understood.

"Do you want to stop the ventilator machine?"

"Yes. I don't want to live that way" was confirmed by repeating the phrase back to her.

"Do you understand that you will die when the ventilator is stopped?"

"Yes."

She said something else I was not sure about. Maybe it was "I want it to be quick."

"Do you know your husband is against your wish?"

"Yes."

"Should we listen to him?"

"No."

"Do you want him included in this decision?"

"No."

I tried to ascertain whether she was legally married. Ms. Barnes "said" that she and her husband were legally married but had been separated for around ten years. Her wishes were clear from this conversation, but I was reluctant to promise a particular outcome. I said she needed to be sure about her decision and that I would speak with Dr. Evans about her wishes.

I began to document the conversation in Ms. Barnes' chart. Then Mr. Barnes phoned the unit to speak with the social worker, Ms. Schultz. I thought about speaking to Mr. Barnes directly, but Ms. Schultz said that he was crying and distraught about the situation – probably not a good time to introduce another person he might see as "against" him. She said Mr. Barnes' opposition seemed to be based on personal issues of his own rather than on his beliefs about his wife's values. Still, he might be moving toward acceptance of his wife's decision.

I completed my lengthy chart note. I recommended that the medical team work with Ms. Barnes as the primary decision-maker to be sure she understood her options and the process of ventilator withdrawal. The doctors were to document the conversations.

When I checked back the following week I saw that Ms. Barnes was still in the hospital on the ventilator. Ms. Czerny did not know whether Dr. Evans had spoken with the patient, but he did say that the family was "dysfunctional." The social worker informed me that Ms. Barnes still refused to consent to nursing home placement and that we could not discharge her against her will. Mr. Barnes continued to have serious emotional problems. I wondered whether someone with these issues could legitimately participate in treatment decisions. Could the hospital recommend counseling? Would Mr. Barnes eventually agree to his wife's request? Why was the healthcare team respecting Ms. Barnes' refusal of nursing home placement but not her wish to stop life-sustaining treatment? Apparently her legal rights did not extend to treatment decisions. The case was becoming more complex. My clear and well-thought-out recommendations had not made any difference. Obviously, I must have done a poor job of consulting. What should I have done differently?

I continued visiting the unit with growing reluctance as the situation remained at an impasse for weeks. Weaning attempts were unsuccessful, Mr. Barnes wanted his wife transferred to a nursing home and he wanted treatment to continue, Ms. Barnes refused to be discharged and wanted to be off the ventilator. We tentatively scheduled an ethics conference to include all those involved in the case, but it was canceled. Nurses became more concerned about the Barneses' relationship. Ms. Barnes' demeanor changed when her husband visited; was he abusive? Someone said there had been an arrest in the family for violence. At times, Mr. Barnes came to the hospital wearing camouflage clothing, and nurses suspected he might have been carrying a knife. Was he a hunter or a member of a paramilitary organization? What, if anything, would this imply about his interactions with others, including his wife? In October the nurses put up Halloween decorations. The cardboard pumpkins, spiders, and witches reminded me of the passage of time, the triviality of death in public awareness, and the real suffering experienced by those in Ms. Barnes' case – a suffering that it seemed I was powerless to change.

Professional reflections

As I look back at this case, I recognize that it was complex, difficult, and could not be resolved by simply identifying and analyzing the dilemma of autonomy vs. paternalism (seemingly based on the wishes of the husband and doctor instead of Ms. Barnes' best interests). Complexities included multiple perspectives among those involved, issues of family dysfunction and emotional instability, perceived threats of violence, worries about lawsuits, uncertainty about the ethics consultation process, logistical problems, and varying power structures within the hospital.

The suffering and vulnerability of Ms. Barnes was buried within this complexity. They were compounded by her ventilator dependence and difficulty communicating. What could have been done differently to improve the outcome? In this case, I would have recommended at least the following:

1. For a new ethics consultant, an in-depth orientation to the clinical setting, which would have included learning the roles and responsibilities of various clinical professionals[1] and working alongside other ethics committee members representing diverse clinical perspectives.[2]
2. Taking the lead in my area of expertise while remaining sensitive and diplomatic. Understanding that shifting perspectives require fluidity of role and analysis.[3]
3. Realizing that the first question asked may not be the most important one but keeping the original requester informed as the case progresses.
4. Providing specific ethical advice in the chart and through direct personal contact. In a Catholic hospital, it is helpful to provide citations from the Ethical and Religious Directives for Catholic Health Care Services.[4]
5. Convening the full ethics committee for review, support, and authority.[5,6]
6. Providing ongoing and persistent follow-up. Making sure that the patient's wishes continue to be explored and heard throughout the hospitalization.
7. Raising the possibility of transfer to another physician.
8. Attempting direct conversation with Mr. Barnes.

Over time I have become more confident in exercising the authority of the ethics committee, and the ethics committee has become better known and respected. We have established policies and procedures for ethics consultation including a reporting form and process for off-hours coverage.

Haunting aspects

There are several haunting aspects to this case. I felt new, inexperienced, and overwhelmed. I doubted my own skills and authority. On the positive side, I tried to attend to all details, including the "classic" stages of ethics consultation (getting permission, careful review of records, speaking with all involved). At the same time, by proceeding so cautiously I might have overlooked opportunities to facilitate an earlier and more ethically sound resolution. I should have been more assertive in gathering information, challenging perspectives, and advocating for the patient herself. The patient eventually agreed to continued support, but was this her authentic decision or did she just get tired of everyone asking? All too often, we assume that when a patient agrees to what "we" think she should do, then the ethical question has been resolved. This consultation should have incorporated more active diplomacy, mediation, and resolution of the various perspectives.

Mr. Barnes remains a shadowy figure. The perception that he was dangerous and intimidating could have been false. If he in fact was dangerous, then security and adult protective services should have been called. I do not know whether this was done. I was worried about my safety, so perhaps I used the social worker's relationship with Mr. Barnes as an excuse to avoid him. Perceiving that the ethical issue was fairly simple, it concerned me that the patient's husband was taking the lead in decisions to the detriment of the patient. I felt – reasonably or not – that I was participating in or condoning a situation that caused her even more suffering.

Another haunting aspect of this case was the look that one of the nurses gave me when Ms. Barnes was being transferred to a "ventilator" extended-care facility. I sensed her expression was accusatory: "Why couldn't you have advocated for this patient and resolved the case?" She said the patient would likely get pneumonia and die because care in the nursing home would not be as skilled. Often when I see that nurse in the hospital, I recall this case and wonder if she remembers it as a bad outcome. Perhaps Ms. Barnes' situation would have been better if my ethics consultation had been more effective. On the other hand, looking back at this early consultation, I recognize that my efforts were a good-faith attempt to change the situation. Relative inexperience in ethics consultation was not the cause of Ms. Barnes' COPD, the dysfunction in her family, or the nurses' frustration. And it is uncertain whether death of the patient, an earlier discharge, or longer survival would have been an improved outcome. Unfortunately, not all the facts and unfolding events are known.

Outcome

Ms. Barnes' hospitalization lasted several more months. She eventually agreed, or became resigned, to remaining on ventilator support, and preparations were made for her discharge to a nursing home. Later I heard that she died several weeks after transfer.

Discussion questions

1. To what extent should ethics consultants allow others to define the process and services of ethics consultation (for example, when one party states that the ethics consultant's recommendations are not needed)?
2. What "powers" do ethics consultants exercise? What are the limitations of these powers? When do we know we have done all that is reasonable to encourage an ethical outcome?
3. How long should the consultant remain involved in a situation when other parties choose not to take recommendations?
4. Identify resources within healthcare settings that can help with complex ethical situations. Which of them might have been useful in the case of Ms. Barnes?
5. What satisfactions do ethics consultants receive from their work? What strategies and resources are useful when an ethics consultant has feelings of failure?

REFERENCES

1. Glover JJ, Nelson W. Innovative educational programs: A necessary first step toward improving quality in ethics consultation. In: Aulisio MP, Arnold RM, Youngner SJ, eds. *Ethics Consultation: From Theory to Practice.* Baltimore, MD: Johns Hopkins; 2003: 53–67.
2. Arnold RM, Wilson Silver MH. Techniques for training ethics consultants: Why traditional classroom methods are not enough. In: Aulisio MP, Arnold RM, Youngner SJ, eds. *Ethics Consultation: From Theory to Practice.* Baltimore: Johns Hopkins; 2003: 70–84.
3. Fletcher JC, Boyle RJ, Spencer EM. Errors in healthcare ethics consultation. In: Rubin SB, Zoloth L, eds. *Margin of Error: The Ethics of Mistakes in the Practice of Medicine.* Hagerstown, MD: University Publishing Group; 2000: 343–72.
4. United States Conference of Catholic Bishops. *Ethical and Religious Directives for Catholic Health Care Services,* 4th ed. Washington, DC: United States Conference of Catholic Bishops, 2001. See, especially, Part 5: Issues in Care for the Dying.
5. Bernal EW. Errors in ethics consultation. In: Rubin SB, Zoloth L, eds. *Margin of Error: The Ethics of Mistakes in the Practice of Medicine.* Hagerstown, MD: University Publishing Group; 2000: 255–72.
6. Rushton C, Youngner SJ, Skeel J. Models for ethics consultation: Individual, team or committee? In: Aulisio MP, Arnold RM, Youngner SJ, eds. *Ethics Consultation: From Theory to Practice.* Baltimore: Johns Hopkins; 2003: 88–94.

14

You're the ethicist; I'm just the surgeon

Joseph P. DeMarco and Paul J. Ford

Case narrative

We did not know what a long day it would be when we first received the call. Joe DeMarco, a visiting scholar from a state university's department of philosophy, was talking with Paul Ford, a bioethicist at a large teaching hospital, about how initial responses were handled for ethics consultations. During this conversation, Paul answered a page. After a brief conversation, he hung up, saying in a perplexed manner that it had been only three days. We quickly left the office, with Joe's initial concern only a reflection of Paul's enigmatic observation, "It's only been three days."

"What do you mean it's only been three days?" Joe asked, not realizing how many times we would hear that phrase over the next eight hours. Paul explained, "It's only been three days since surgery, and the family wants the patient removed from life support." Paul looked pensive; perhaps "worried" is too strong.

The consultation was initiated by Nurse Abigail, who was caring for the patient at bedside. However, the actual consult page came from the intensivist, Dr. Bryan.

Nurse Abigail told us her concern about the patient's suffering and about the family's wishes related to discontinuing life-sustaining treatment being ignored. Clearly, the circumstances upset her; she seemed somewhat angry. That was tempered by her respect for, maybe fear of, the patient's surgeon.

Mr. Carl, a 60-year-old man, had open-heart surgery three days prior. He had multiple medical problems, including kidney failure. He required continuous ventilator support through the entire postoperative course, and Mrs. Carl reported that he only occasionally communicated. She claimed that Mr. Carl was in significant pain and great discomfort. Nevertheless, he lay nearly motionless in bed. Nurse Abigail indicated that the surgeon, Dr. Dallas, had been unwilling to withdraw the ventilator.

Mrs. Carl was agitated when we first saw her. She had been demanding that the ventilator be withdrawn. She may have been receiving moral support from the

nurses on this point. Mrs. Carl felt that she fully understood Mr. Carl's circumstances. She and Mr. Carl had frequently communicated about facing a low quality
of life due to illness, and she knew that Mr. Carl would not consent to being on a
ventilator.

Mrs. Carl's agitation was compounded by the fact that she was from out of state,
staying at a local hotel. She complained that the delay in removing the ventilator
would soon cause her to miss the hotel's checkout time and force her to stay an
extra day.

Paul soon talked with Dr. Dallas by phone. Dr. Dallas spoke in a professional
manner but let Paul know he was not pleased about the ethics consultation.
"It was only three days since the surgery. What did they expect?" His integrity
seemed on the line. He obviously took pride in his abilities as a surgeon and in
his willingness to take on a difficult case. According to the surgeon, the patient
understood prior to the surgery that the outcome was unsure. In fact, Dr. Dallas
was sure that everyone understood this before the surgery, including the patient's
wife. Although he insisted that he knew the right thing to do in cases like these, he
would not object to having bioethics present during the family meeting. Believing
that a bioethics presence would facilitate a consensus, Paul accepted this tenuous
invitation.

In the meantime, after careful consideration Dr. Bryan (the intensivist who
initiated the consult) decided to determine whether Mr. Carl could survive without
the ventilator. If the patient did not need the ventilator, then the withdrawal would
be a moot point. He ordered the oxygen levels to be gradually reduced over the
next few minutes while carefully observing Mr. Carl's condition. We watched as
the test began: Mr. Carl, for the first time, clearly moved and made some unusual
sounds. The few minutes seemed protracted and were difficult to witness.

Nurse Abigail walked away from the bed space as the test was underway. As she
passed by, she angrily but quietly said the ventilator test was cruel and immoral.
Could it be immoral? Did our actions lead to it? To Joe, the whole situation seemed
to be from a TV movie, with someone writing an improbable script.

It soon became clear that Mr. Carl would not survive off the ventilator. The test
ended and the ventilator settings were returned to their previous levels. This simply
reinstated the temporarily forgotten impending dilemma concerning withdrawal
of this therapy.

A couple of hours later, we met with Nurse Abigail, Mrs. Carl, Mr. Carl's adult
son, Dr. Dallas, and Dr. Bryan.

The meeting began with Dr. Dallas making observations about the case. He
talked in a friendly but authoritarian manner about the case as he saw it. It was
too soon, he thought, to "give up" on Mr. Carl. Even though Dr. Dallas admitted
that the chances of recovery were slim, he asked for a few more days to be sure
Mr. Carl was not going to regain his health.

Mrs. Carl firmly but politely rejected Dr. Dallas' statement and request. She said
her husband would not approve of being ventilator dependent and that he had

previously made his wishes clear. The son, in a less assertive way, expressed full agreement. Mrs. Carl believed Mr. Carl would not want to be ventilator dependent even for a few hours, which she quickly changed to a few days. Simply stated, the surgery had not gone as well as they had hoped, and it was now time to stop.

Dr. Dallas seemed surprised at Mrs. Carl's insistence that the ventilator be removed, perhaps thinking that his opening statement was reasonable and well enough performed so Mrs. Carl would allow continuation of the current level of treatment. Dr. Dallas became less friendly and more challenging. He told Mrs. Carl that Mr. Carl had been fully aware of the risks. He had understood recovery would not be easy, but he wanted to try it anyway. Dr. Dallas was under the impression that Mr. Carl would not have wanted to give up after only three days.

Maybe Dr. Dallas thought there was an implicit agreement that consenting to surgery involved consenting to the difficulties of the recovery period. In all likelihood, he would not have performed the surgery had he been told that therapy would be withdrawn this quickly. Mrs. Carl did not deny Dr. Dallas' account of the presurgery meeting. But she insisted that Mr. Carl had been heavily drugged at the time and was not able to state his long-standing view of ventilators and quality of life. Dr. Dallas rejected this, repeating Mr. Carl's words from that meeting, "Let's give it a try." Dr. Dallas thought that three days did not constitute a "try"; Mrs. Carl thought that the "try" had failed.

Mrs. Carl was done talking. Her tone changed dramatically. She was angry and insisted that it was her legal right to make decisions for her husband and she wanted the ventilator removed. No more aggressive interventions would be approved. At this, Dr. Dallas backed down. He indicated that he would not stand in the way. He was then paged and left the room, as did the family and Nurse Abigail.

Dr. Bryan was displeased with this outcome. He was concerned that the ventilation was at a low level; the patient's need for oxygen was not nearly as high as he had observed in many similar patients. He repeated, perhaps as many as four times, "But the oxygen requirements are low." Medical opinion was fairly clear: It was too early to make a prognosis, to give up on Mr. Carl. After all, it had only been three days.

Dr. Dallas re-entered, saying to the three of us: "She [Mrs. Carl] just wants him zipped up in a body bag." There was no response from anyone in the room. Then his tone changed. He wanted to know whether he was doing the right thing. He could not order the ventilator removed – that would be going too far for him. But he would not stand in the way of this being done by others. Did this amount to the same thing? Was he abandoning his patient? Was he doing the right thing? He faced his own moral dilemma.

Joe observed the interchange between Paul and Dr. Dallas. Amazing! Dr. Dallas went from the person who knew the right thing to do to a medical professional facing a genuine moral dilemma – a problem that obviously confounded him. It is easy to know the right thing to do when everything goes as planned and there is no conflict or opposition. However, the current case was not easy.

The dialogue became more amazing. Dr. Dallas said, in a troubled way, "I'm only a surgeon. I don't know about ethics. You're an ethicist. You know. Am I doing the right thing? It feels like I am abandoning this patient." Joe thought that Dr. Dallas was looking for consolation, comfort, or maybe even absolution, but not really for ethical knowledge. Paul responded without emotional affect, seemingly understanding that Dr. Dallas was requesting information much like a student requests information in a class. Paul affirmed that Dr. Dallas had clearly stated his view to Mrs. Carl, that Dr. Dallas was respecting the wishes of the family and thus was respecting informed consent through a proxy decision-maker by allowing the withdrawal of therapy. Paul's clear and thorough reply apparently satisfied Dr. Dallas.

We had been on the case for almost nine hours. We stood close to Mr. Carl's bed for many of them, only seeing part of his face. He seemed almost unreal after awhile except for the brief weaning trial. As we approached the bed after the family meeting, Mr. Carl seemed more like a living person with a real history. This made the situation feel tougher. We understood that the deliberations were over and that a living person would soon die.

Nurse Abigail received the orders for withdrawal. Mrs. Carl remained at bedside to provide whatever comfort was possible for her husband. Her son left the bedside. Just before the process started, Paul asked Mrs. Carl if she wanted clergy present. She declined. We soon left with Mr. Carl still breathing.

It was difficult to sleep that night. It took much reflection to pinpoint the most troubling issues.

Professional reflections

It is easy to challenge the authority of a bioethicist. Dr. Dallas, in his own way, did exactly that at the outset of the case. Suppose Dr. Dallas is correct, that he knows better about this situation than everyone else. Suppose that he does not need help. He is, after all, an experienced surgeon who probably best knows the medical condition of the patient. He discussed the surgery with the patient; we had not. Can the bioethicist do more harm than good? What is the bioethicist's role? What would it be in this case? If there is some type of "authority," where does it arise from?

By the end of the case, the surgeon looked to bioethics for help. Joe thought about whether it would have been better to offer words of comfort to the surgeon at the end. But those would not have lasted and could have been empty. Paul explained the justification for the decisions being made. That type of explanation was one that could last.

Often ethics is presented in terms of making the right decision. However, in a moral dilemma, there is a conflict over values. A final decision means that one value "wins" over the others.[1] There is a genuine loss of value. If circumstances were different in the case, all values may be able to be preserved. Dr. Dallas lost in terms of valuation of his professional judgment of what's best for this patient. We can only wonder about the repercussions to him. Professional conscience was bound to be compromised. Nurse Abigail was even more adamant. Had the case been further lengthened, she would have suffered her own loss because of her perception of injustice and harm being done. We lost the hope of achieving a full consensus that would have helped assuage the haunting character of the case.

If Dr. Dallas had insisted on extra time, then that might have compromised Mr. Carl's autonomy, possibly leaving him with pain and suffering that his wife claimed he would have avoided by rejecting treatment. We might have violated the concern and care of his wife and son.

Haunting aspects

We do not need to know people personally to be haunted by their deaths. Witnessing the dying process itself is sometimes haunting. But it was more than simply death or sadness in this case. We participated in decision making that directly led to a person's death. If not for that process, there is a significant chance that Mr. Carl would be alive today. We did not make the decision; Dr. Dallas did. But that is not a fair statement. Dr. Dallas did not want to concede to Mrs. Carl. It seemed as though he was suspicious of her motivation, felt an affront to his professional integrity, and wanted to see the patient survive. All things considered, he did not believe "giving up" after only three days was reasonable. Had he received support for his position from someone else at that family meeting, he may not have stepped aside and allowed the withdrawal. He surely knew he had options that would buy time, such as seeking legal intervention to have a guardian declared. He did not do these things. The presence of an ethicist influenced the surgeon's behavior. After all, no one in the room offered support for Dr. Dallas' position. Without an ally, he may have defaulted to the wife's demands.

We could have recommended ways to give Mr. Carl more time. We did not. The fact that we did not make the decision does not absolve us. We made our decision not to support Dr. Dallas, not to question Mrs. Carl's motivations, and not to ask for more time. Mr. Carl's poor medical condition, his wife's firm statements, and his son's acquiescence all pointed to a legitimate, albeit inconclusive, rejection of aggressive treatment. It was haunting to participate in this person's death, whether right or wrong. Similarly, the bioethicist's explanation of ethical permissibility and obligation did not absolve Dr. Dallas from his responsibilities. However, it may have provided him a context and support for that which was lost.

Morality is not simply a matter of opinion. A bioethicist can be wrong.[2] We could have been wrong in this case. If we were, a person would have died without the chance he should have had. In this case, we relied on the substituted judgment of Mrs. Carl. She presented in detail that Mr. Carl would not want the current therapy. There is ample reason to suspect that Mrs. Carl had a conflict of interest.[3,4] Maybe there was a financial conflict. Maybe future caring for her husband was hard for her to bear. Maybe he was far from the ideal father and husband, someone whose death would be welcomed. If it had only been Mrs. Carl, we probably would have more strongly suspected a conflict. But her views were corroborated by her son, who seemed more concerned about Mr. Carl. Further, a daughter living in another state also supported the decision. However, such corroboration is not conclusive. There may be unknown conflicts of interest that could invalidate the whole family's decision. These may have tainted the family's judgments. After all, Mr. Carl told the surgeon that he wanted to give the surgery a chance. We had no way to acquire complete knowledge of the case. Were we right?

At best, bioethics is an unsettled discipline. Having a standard of practice is consoling because it means that a good deal of agreement exists about the right thing to do. With such, one does not stand alone. We stood in this case without such support. What would another bioethicist have done? Would the outcome have been different? Would Mr. Carl be alive today? Did we unduly influence the case in one direction?

If we had not been supportive of Mrs. Carl's rights, maybe Mrs. Carl and her son would have agreed to give Mr. Carl a few more days. Maybe Mr. Carl may have been able to communicate his own desires a day later, reducing the chance of making the moral error of ending a fight for life that was desired. We did not dissolve the dilemma. Had that happened, the case may not have been as haunting.

Mr. Carl's death gives us reason to strive for more professionalism in bioethics with clearer standards of practice and more agreement among consultants. Dr. Dallas' statement persists, "You're the ethicist; I'm just a surgeon." He thought of us as having consultative expertise in the realm of ethics. Given this expectation, we as a discipline need to continue to develop our skills and competencies to provide the best quality advice possible.

Outcome

The next morning we checked the electronic medical record. Mr. Carl died sometime between 7 p.m. and midnight of the same day we consulted. We had no further follow-up.

Discussion questions

1. Mrs. Carl wanted the deliberations to go quickly so she wouldn't have to spend an additional day in the hotel. Does the desire to leave suggest a conflict of interest for a proxy?

2. Was there a need for a proxy decision? That is, did Mr. Carl's initial consent still hold or had conditions changed enough to require ongoing consent?
3. How do you think Dr. Dallas would have acted without the presence of bioethics?
4. Nurse Abigail protested that the test to determine whether Mr. Carl could be weaned from the ventilator was immoral? Was she right?
5. Does it make sense to talk about "moral error" in this case? Does it involve a judgment call that is neither right nor wrong?

REFERENCES

1. DeMarco JP, Ford PJ. Balancing in ethical deliberation: Superior to specification and casuistry. *J Med Philos*, 2006; 31(5): 483–97.
2. Bernal E. Errors in ethics consultation. In: Rubin SB, Zoloth L, eds. *Margin of Error: The Ethics of Mistakes in the Practice of Medicine.* Hagerstown, MD: University Publishing Group; 2000: 255–72.
3. Hardwig J. The problem of proxies with interests of their own: Toward a better theory of proxy decisions. *J Clin Ethics*, 1993; 4(1): 20–7.
4. Brody BA. Hardwig on proxy decision making. *J Clin Ethics*, 1993; 4(1): 66–7.

15

Haunted by a good outcome: the case of Sister Jane

George J. Agich

Case narrative

The patient, whom I will call Sister Jane, is a 70-year-old Roman Catholic nun with a living will and power of attorney for health care naming another nun as her agent. She is in the cardiac surgical intensive-care unit after a mitral valve replacement and coronary artery bypass surgery performed emergently after a myocardial infarction. She has a history of coronary artery disease, hypertension, and a 50-pack-per-year history of smoking. Postoperative complications included acute renal failure, respiratory failure, and a pseudomonas sepsis. The patient is currently on a ventilator with a tracheostomy. The sepsis is improving. Sister Jane has been unusually oppositional and troublesome throughout her stay. Nurses describe her as a demanding patient whose postsurgical complications were rough. Nuns from her convent corroborated that Sister Jane's attitude was "difficult and challenging" in the best of circumstances.

During one of the regular ethics liaison rounds,[1] the critical-care physician requested a formal ethics consultation because the patient had asked that all treatments be stopped. Although she had refused to cooperate with treatment in the past, these refusals were judged to be part of a difficult postoperative adjustment. When her treatment opposition was discussed with her on previous occasions, she admitted being despondent. She attributed her despondency to the difficult recovery, but in each instance she eventually accepted the treatments. At these times, Sister Jane was told she had the right to refuse life support if the treatment was more than she could bear. Despite a continuing pattern of being difficult to care for and uncooperative, Sister Jane always declined to stop or otherwise limit ongoing treatment. The critical-care physician asked me to review Sister Jane's request since, at this time, the surgical and critical-care teams both judged that she was now clearly unwilling to continue treatment. I was informed that this

The author extends his special thanks to his research assistant, Vassiliki Leontis, for important editorial suggestions.

was ethically troubling to the critical-care and surgical teams because the patient's sepsis and her strength were improving to the point where she could begin to be weaned from the ventilator. Nevertheless, both teams acknowledged and accepted the patient's right to refuse treatment. They requested that I review and validate this course of action.

The formal ethics consultation began with the critical-care physician characterizing the ethical problem as "Sister Jane's refusal of life-sustaining treatment in the face of improvement in her underlying condition." He stated that the patient wanted the ventilator stopped. He said that even though she was told that doing so would result in her death, she persisted. The critical-care physician reported that her reaction to being told about her improving condition was tearful and that the critical-care team had observed increasing anxiety since the discussion. He also stated that Sister Jane appeared to be depressed during the last two days and that early in her stay he had discussed with the surgeon trying antidepressant medication, but Sister Jane became septic and required sedation instead. The critical-care physician said he hoped that "reducing her dependence on the ventilator [would] . . . improve her mental status and attitude towards removing life support." I questioned this proposition. He responded that we would never know because psychiatry consultation had been offered to address her depression and to help deal with the strain of treatment, but she had refused. Her sepsis was almost fully resolved.

Given the patient's improving status and her clear communication that she wanted life support removed, the following ethical question was put to me: "Does the patient have decisional capacity to insist that she be withdrawn from the ventilator since she is not terminally ill?" I was informed about the patient's difficult postoperative course, which her physicians thought could explain her decision to "call it quits." In their progress notes, the surgeon and critical-care physician wrote that they "were willing to commence withdrawing the ventilator if the patient persisted in her request to do so, but only after appropriate ethics review." With this background, I interviewed the patient.

At the interview, Sister Jane communicated by mouthing words and writing responses. The bedside critical-care nurse's assistance was invaluable in the interpretation. Sister Jane indicated that she understood my role and welcomed my involvement. I accepted this as permission to proceed and did not seek additional consent. Sister Jane corroborated the difficult course of her treatment in the intensive-care unit. She also acknowledged that she was "unwilling and unable to continue [it]." By asking questions about her medical situation, the cause of her illness, and the outcome of her surgery and prognosis, I confirmed that her comprehension of her situation was accurate. Her facial expression lacked emotion, to be sure, but she displayed a thorough understanding of her dependence on the ventilator for respiratory support. She readily acknowledged feeling depressed but attributed this feeling to her prolonged physical suffering. As to the offer of psychiatric consultation, she said she was unwilling to be seen by a psychiatrist. She also indicated that she was ready to die but wanted no action taken to remove her from the ventilator until her decision was discussed with her mother superior and her healthcare agent the next day.

I asked Sister Jane if she would allow a psychiatrist to confirm her decisional ability. I told her that both her physicians and I accepted that she has the capacity to make decisions for herself, but since terminating life support is such an important decision, we would appreciate a psychiatrist's corroboration. She refused to see the psychiatrist. If her decisional ability were judged to be lacking at this point, her advance directives could come into play, she pointed out to me, a point that I also acknowledged. The next day the bedside nurse reported that after my interview some nuns visited. They learned about Sister Jane's request to have the ventilator withdrawn and expressed personal support for this decision.

The case evolved over several days during which Sister Jane accepted all interventions. Nonetheless, she planned and prayed with the nuns, who increased their visits with her. She continued to want the ventilator stopped. Finally, she arranged one last visit with the nuns. At that time she and they expected that life support would be withdrawn.

I was called to the unit to join a meeting the next morning involving the mother superior, Sister Jane's healthcare agent, some other nuns, the surgical fellow, and the critical-care physician. At my arrival, discussion about the process of disconnecting the ventilator was in progress. The decision to withdraw life support seemed to be clear to everyone at the meeting. I stated that even though everyone accepted Sister Jane's right to refuse treatment, I was troubled by the ambiguity in her communication and decision making. The critical-care physician stated that the paradoxical character of her request to stop life support just as she was improving led to the request for ethical review of the case. The nuns also admitted that Sister Jane gave "mixed messages" about her wishes. After leading a discussion on the ethical responsibility of ensuring the soundness of the patient's decision making, I suggested that a bedside interview be conducted with Sister Jane to address these lingering concerns. As the group proceeded to her bedside, it was agreed that I should lead the discussion with the patient since I had by this time directly communicated with her about removing life support more than other caregivers had.

At the bedside, I told Sister Jane that the entire group around her bed acknowledged the difficult time she had in the critical-care unit and that everyone supported her right to refuse life support. However, because the decision to remove the ventilator was so ethically significant, I said I needed to ask again not only what she wanted done, but why. She pointed to the tracheostomy, indicating that she wanted it removed, and everyone at the bedside, except me, interpreted this to mean that she wanted the ventilator removed. The nun, who was her healthcare agent, expressed this aloud. Yet her gesture as she looked at me raised a doubt in my mind that prompted me to ask whether it was the tracheostomy or the ventilator that she wanted removed. At this question, she looked quite confused. She asked "Aren't they same?"

The bedside nurse interjected that they had repeatedly told Sister Jane the tracheostomy was essential to maintain respiratory support. The critical-care physician looked at me with an expression of insight. He then explained to Sister Jane that although the tracheostomy was essential for assisting with her respiration, addressing a problem with the tracheostomy (if there were one) might not require stopping life support. He said he wondered whether her difficulty with the tracheostomy was related to the relatively large-diameter tube that was placed during the original resuscitation and intubation. He said he wondered if her frustration and discomfort were more related to the tube, which he said they could address, than to the ventilator. He offered her the option of removing the tracheostomy tube and replacing it with a smaller-diameter, vented tube that might be more comfortable and would allow her to block the vent, enabling her to speak. The nuns reacted positively to this new information, but Sister Jane seemed wary and noncommittal. I asked whether she had additional problems, and she said the critical-care unit was uncomfortable. "Too much noise, too much activity, not a moment of peace, even at night. I can't sleep." The critical-care physician promised that he could solve this problem by changing her nighttime medication, which would give her a solid night's sleep.

I confirmed that she had no other reason for insisting that life support be stopped other than discomfort with the tracheostomy and her inability to sleep through the night. I asked if she wanted to try having the tracheostomy changed and her medication altered to help her sleep. I stressed that she would still have the right to refuse life support and asked the critical-care physician to explain to her (and the nuns) what was involved in revising the tracheostomy before she made a decision. Following these explanations, Sister Jane held up two fingers indicating that she would accept this plan on the condition that these actions improve her condition in just two days.

This unexpected outcome seemed to please everyone, and the bedside meeting ended. The physician and surgical fellow stated as they left the bedside that there was no (medical or surgical) reason for her to be allowed to die. I reminded them that her right to refuse treatment was not limited by their medical assessment. They both agreed and expressed their happiness that I had uncovered new treatment options. Later that day the cardiac surgeon called me to say that he appreciated the new "treatment plan." He said it gave him a new appreciation of what clinical ethics consultation can accomplish! The plan was implemented with success. A few days later, Sister Jane was transferred to a hospital closer to her convent for continued weaning from the ventilator. She subsequently sent a letter to the critical-care unit thanking the staff for its care and for tolerating her stubbornness.

Professional reflections

This case provides a cautionary tale about the complexity of ethics consultation and the responsibility of ethics consultants. It warns that it is all-too-easy for ethics consultants to tacitly accept an obvious ethical problem as presented. Accepting a problem or issue *as it is defined* for ethics consultants at a particular moment in the evolution of a patient's care as *the* ethical problem is highly questionable. This case raises the following questions: Should consultants simply address the questions presented to them and completely leave the management of the case in the hands of physicians (and other health professionals) who are responsible for the care of the patient? Is it appropriate for the ethics consultant to take on a "management" function through communications and recommendations that affect the circumstances and outcomes of a case or to simply validate a predefined course of action?

Becoming involved in ongoing cases raises a series of boundary issues about the actions and recommendations that ethics consultants may appropriately make and whether independent actions are appropriate (and if so, what type). A corollary question is the degree to which ethics consultants should rely on, without further investigation or corroboration, the so-called clinical facts of the case, which inevitably structure the ethical issues.

In this case, a routine question was posed to an ethics consultant. Hospital policy and the legal framework for withdrawing life support were clearly understood. Neither required the involvement of ethics consultation in such decisions. Normally, if there is no conflict, treatment abatement occurs without ethics consultation. In this case, ethics consultation was requested to validate the decision making. In some settings, ethical review of a case and validation occur at some distance from the patient-care setting. This oversight involves phone conversations, ethics committee or consultative team meetings, review of the medical record, and the entering of a summary note or report documenting approval of, or concurrence with, the decision. In cases where there is ambivalence or concern about some aspect of the situation, ethics consultants are likely to be more closely involved in the case and to interact directly with the principal parties. Although the ethical question was whether Sister Jane was competent to refuse life support, the circumstances of her ambivalence and the ambiguity of some of her communications raised sufficient doubt in the mind of the critical-care physician. This brought about the ethics consultation. Practically, however, the way out of the impasse was to turn to the healthcare agent – as Sister Jane pointed out – who in this case supported the decision to withdraw life support. Since the surgical and critical-care teams, healthcare agent, and nuns all accepted Sister Jane's right to refuse life support, it would have been easy to validate that the decision making was ethically sound. Such a validation, however, could have been based on a thin understanding of what was on closer inspection a complex request. My interactions with Sister Jane challenged me to be open to other interpretations and options.

This case raises a cautionary flag that ethical problems as they are presented need to be assessed with due care by ethics consultants. I took the lead at the bedside interview, which may raise questions about the boundary and limits of the ethics consultant's role. Given the wider context of critical-care liaison rounds, which framed this consultation request, a collaborative and engaged role was understandable. This case, however, makes the general point that ethics consultants, like all individuals and professionals, are prone to mistakenly accepting matters as defined by others. The ethical issue presented initially in this case was a refusal of life-sustaining treatment, which I was asked to validate. However, accepting this interpretation without further investigation would have pushed the case in a direction that might have been disastrous.

Haunting aspects

This case warns about the alleged "culture of death" that Wesley J. Smith has charged is a tacit feature of liberal bioethics.[2] While his view is not well argued or established for bioethics in general, his criticism underscores a vexing question that *should* haunt all ethics consultants: To what extent do "easy" or "routine" end-of-life cases receive an uncritical or routine handling that uncritically incorporates acceptance of death?[3] To what extent do ethics consultants function in an institutional and social framework that takes for granted the protection of the patient's right to refuse life-sustaining treatment in ways that *promote* refusal? This case is haunting not because of its bad outcome, but because it pointedly asks: To what extent is ethics consultation part of the "culture of death?" Did the patient's religion, which accepts the natural and inevitable passing with the hope of a reunion with God, or Sister Jane's spiritual maturity influence our acceptance of the case as an "end-of-life" dilemma?

If ethics consultants see themselves as primarily involved in "end-of-life decision making," they will tend to view their cases from the perspective of a "culture of death." Given the history of the field, this seems to be a fundamental tendency of many ethics consultants. The capacity to view the case afresh and to identify latent problems, however, is the greatest contribution ethics consultants can bring to ethically complex cases. This is a challenging and potentially elusive goal that requires ethics consultants to accept the responsibilities associated with this goal. Despite reinforcements to the contrary, ethics consultations should never be performed in a perfunctory or routine fashion. Ethics consultants need to pay close attention to the details of every case and to regard critically the interpretations offered to them. Otherwise, any of us might fail to recognize other Sister Janes among the patients with whom we consult.

Discussion questions

1. What should an "appropriate ethics review" as requested by the critical-care physician involve?
2. To what extent should medical options be suggested by an ethics consultant?
3. Do ethics consultants need to explicitly ask a patient for permission to undertake an ethics consultation? If they refuse, is there still a role for the consultant?
4. How do we avoid promoting "withdrawal" and avoid rubber-stamping decisions?

REFERENCES

1. Agich GJ. Joining the team: Ethics consultation at the Cleveland Clinic. *HEC Forum*, 2003; 15(4): 310–22.
2. Smith WJ. *Culture of Death: The Assault on Medical Ethics in America.* San Francisco: Encounter Books, 2000.
3. Wynia MK, Derse A. Book review: Culture of death: The assault on medical ethics in America. *Medsc Gen Med*, 2001; 3(3).

16

Is a broken jaw a terminal condition?

Stuart G. Finder

Case narrative

The request for ethics consultation came from the trauma unit charge nurse on a Friday afternoon. My secretary, using the "Request for Consultation Information Form" my colleague and I developed, took the call. This form has space to list basic facts, including "Patient history, situation, and prognosis." It also contains two key questions, the answers to which are to be written verbatim. First, "What is the reason for this call?" Second, "What does the caller hope to accomplish with this inquiry?"

From the form I learned the patient, Mary Jackson, was an 83-year-old recent widow in a step-down bed in the trauma unit. The reason for the call was, "The patient is DNR [do not resuscitate], but the physicians have decided to put her back on oxygen." As for what the charge nurse hoped would be accomplished, my secretary had written, "Was it ethical for the doctor to order oxygen for the patient?" Under "Patient history, situation, and prognosis" was this:

Patient had auto accident earlier in week. Fractured jaw & broken elbow. Pt has dementia. Daughter doesn't want anything done. No surgery to her jaw and was taken off oxygen. Has Do Not Resuscitate (DNR). Attending put her back on oxygen because she was struggling to breathe. Nurses feel she would be fine with surgery and food (taken off food because she was scheduled for surgery) in a nursing home.

Review of Mrs. Jackson's electronic record revealed she was admitted on Monday after sustaining a variety of minor orthopedic injuries – fractured right wrist, dislocated right elbow, broken right rib, and mandible fracture – as the result of her single-vehicle accident. Her only other injury was a 4-cm laceration over her right cheek. Nothing in her past medical history, including mild dementia, was noted as contributing to her accident.

I also learned that by Wednesday evening her laceration had been closed, her arm injuries had been repaired, and fixation of her jaw fracture was scheduled for Thursday. However, Thursday morning she went into respiratory distress and was intubated. Although she was extubated by day's end, the oral surgeons postponed her surgery indefinitely and Gregg McCord, the attending trauma surgeon, wrote a DNR order. In his accompanying note he referred to Mrs. Jackson as "a woman with a poor quality of life following injury and arrest." He arranged to meet with her daughter and son-in-law (Marcia and Doug Elam) the following morning to discuss care options.

That meeting took place a few hours before ethics consultation was requested.

Dr. McCord, case manager Linda Kelly, and social worker Jean Brightman documented the discussion with the Elams, who expressed concern about Mrs. Jackson's condition and her preference. The Elams said that during her husband's long illness, Mrs. Jackson said she would not want long-term nursing home care. Dr. McCord wrote that "the patient requires extensive surgery, placement of a feeding tube, and subsequent convalescent care," while Ms. Kelly noted that Mrs. Elam said she would be unable to care for her mother at home. Ms. Brightman noted Mrs. Elam "expressed concern about her mother's declining mental status."

With all of this in mind and more questions than answers – why, for instance, was there such a negative outlook regarding Mrs. Jackson's prognosis; there seemed to be a gap in the narrative – I set off for the trauma unit. I wondered whether the nurses, too, had sensed that gap, but it hadn't been mentioned. Instead, the request focused on reinitiating oxygen support after implementing the DNR. What was going on?

Once in the trauma unit, I spoke briefly with Connie, the charge nurse who had made the request, Sara, the bedside nurse, Linda Kelly, and finally Jean Brightman. While both Connie and Sara mentioned the oxygen and DNR issue, each quickly shifted to the broader question of why surgery was not being pursued. Ms. Kelly and Ms. Brightman expressed concern that Mrs. Elam was making the "wrong" choice.

In fact, Ms. Brightman told me she was skeptical of the daughter's intentions. "This woman and her husband seemed disinterested," she said in reference to their meeting earlier. "I mean, after we'd just decided to withdraw care, she gets out her cell phone and calls a friend to see where to meet for lunch when the meeting is over. This isn't what you do right after you've made this kind of decision." But she had, and the Elams had left the hospital to meet their friends. They had yet to return, and Sara told me they were not answering their cell phone.

I would have liked to talk with Mrs. Jackson, but she was just sitting in her room, breathing heavily, staring off. She barely moved and did not respond to anything Sara said. I left the unit. It still seemed odd that emphasis was now going to shift to palliation. There *had* to be something else going on. Mrs. Jackson said she would not want *long-term* placement in a nursing home, but was that *really* what she was facing?

I spoke with Dr. McCord a few hours later by phone. He had no qualms about the decision to limit interventions. He told me of several conversations with Mrs. Elam. She had been staying in the hospital around the clock, had readily consented to whatever he suggested was necessary, and seemed genuinely concerned about her mother's situation. She struck him as a very loving and devoted daughter who was simply trying to do what was best for her mother. "And," he said, "this isn't as simple a case as it seems."

Specifically: "While fixing the mandible is straightforward enough, recovery is going to be taxing. She'll require full-time nursing support for at least several months, which her daughter can't provide and her insurance won't cover if done at home. So that means nursing home placement. For that, she'll need a PEG (percutaneous endoscopic gastrostomy feeding tube) because no facility will accept an 83-year-old woman with diminished capacity and a wired-shut jaw without one. And truth be told, she'll need it; I don't think she has the ability otherwise to take in enough calories to heal well. And you know, she's likely to get pneumonia soon enough, then we'll be looking at a tracheostomy. And, she doesn't even *want* to go to a nursing home."

He also noted her recovery would be stressful and would likely "push her over the edge" so that she would end up nursing home dependent for the long term. Plus, elderly patients in nursing homes with trachs and PEGs often do not do well. "The option is fix her jaw and condemn her to the nursing home and a slow death or keep her comfortable and allow her to die with some dignity."

"What's the deal with the nasal cannula?" I asked. This *was* the issue I had been called about. He said he viewed oxygen as a comfort measure, a better option than morphine, which may calm her but would also make her unable to interact with her daughter. I heard his pager go off, then he told me he had to go. He thanked me for the call and hung up.

Things now seemed both simplified and more complex. I could appreciate Dr. McCord's perspective, especially if his report of the daughter's concerns was accurate. But why had the others – nurses, case manager, social worker – come away with such a different picture? Were they imposing their own preconceptions and expectations, or was this physician misreading matters? To find out I headed back to the unit to tell the nurses what I had learned.

I discovered that Mrs. Elam had not returned or called, and there were even more nurses who were concerned. Several came over when I began to tell Connie what I had learned. They *all* had discussed this, and *no one* agreed with the plan not to repair Mrs. Jackson's jaw. They listened closely to my report. When I was through, several shook their heads and gave me a "that makes sense" look, but most did not. "I can understand that," one said, "but I still think it's wrong. After all, *if* it's accurate she said she didn't want to end up in a nursing home, she was discussing this as her husband was dying. I don't think that's the best time to be making decisions – while your husband is dying." Others agreed.

Another went further. "This poor lady's been through hell watching her husband die. She needs time to recover. And I bet the daughter's worn out, too, maybe even too worn out to care at the moment. I don't mean to be judgmental, but I'd never treat my mother this way." There was some underlying anger in her voice, and several nurses seemed to share it. Then she said, "But she's not my patient, I'm just the nurse, and if McCord can live with this, then . . ." and her voice trailed off.

There was a natural break in the discussion. Connie seemed relieved, and she thanked me. I had apparently done what she wanted, although *I* did not feel any clearer. In fact, I was more unsettled. I had discovered just enough to feel the distress of these nurses – and there was really very little I could do. Was that it then? Was the consult now over? I may have thought so, but I was wrong.

The next day, Saturday, I was paged around 3:30 p.m. by the administrator on call. She wanted to talk about what had happened with Mrs. Jackson.

Mrs. Jackson's new nurse had refused a phone order from Dr. McCord to discontinue the oxygen and start a midazolam-fentanyl drip. The nurse disagreed with that plan, so he went to his assistant manager and told her he would not comply. She called the administrator on call, who came to the unit and with the assistant manager took over Mrs. Jackson's care. This was around 11:00 a.m. They administered a small bolus of morphine before removing the nasal cannula. Then they started the drip. Mrs. Jackson died around 2:30 p.m. Although she had been told what was occurring, Mrs. Elam did not come in. The staff was really bothered, and the administrator on call debriefed them. Now *she* was having second thoughts and was overcome with doubt. She called me because she hoped I could confirm she had "done the right thing."

As I listened to her story, I wondered the same, although not about her. I wondered whether *I* had done the right thing, whether *I* had pursued the issues far enough. I had never spoken with Mrs. Elam, had not followed up with Dr. McCord, had not checked in with Saturday's nurses. What responsibility did I now bear for Mrs. Jackson's death?

If I had been uncertain and unsettled the day before, I was even more so today.

Professional reflections

The issue of responsibility in clinical ethics consultation, and more particularly the *experience of feeling, and hence "being" responsible* in a real and specific patient-care situation, has not received much attention in clinical ethics literature. But in practice the issue of responsibility is always present. In the situation involving Mrs. Jackson it was, in many senses, the core issue – for the nurses, Dr. McCord, the Elams, the administrator on call, and me. From my own confrontation with this issue, a few brief points may be noted.

First and foremost, whatever method of ethics consultation is pursued entails talking with others who, to some degree or another, face choices, decisions, or outcomes that raise questions about what they hold valuable and worthwhile.[1] But as my interactions in this situation reveal, it is not always explicitly clear just what those values are, let alone which choice, decision, or outcome is *most* worthwhile.

Moreover, it is not merely the values of those others that may be at stake as well as hidden or unclear; the same holds true for me as I try to identify, clarify, and articulate the choices, decisions, and outcomes most consonant with what those primary decision-makers hold to be most worthwhile and willing and able to enact.[2] Plus, engaging others about such matters is not benign; what I say or do – for instance, how I respond to the administrator on call – can influence and even change how those others understand their choices and decisions.[3]

Clinical ethics responsibility, therefore, demands that ethics consultants be responsive to what those individuals indicate as *their* concerns as well as "*explicitly and deliberately take on or assume* the responsibility for" what subsequently unfolds when identifying various options, clarifying likely choices and decisions, and articulating the possibly multiple meanings associated with potential outcomes.[4] Part and parcel with such responsibility is thus the real possibility that the ethics consultant confronts an ever-present possibility for error[2] – in this case, such an error may have contributed to Mrs. Jackson's death.

The question of my responsibility in Mrs. Jackson's death, then, like all questions of responsibility in the practice of clinical ethics consultation, is no mere theoretical or academic wondering. It reflects the experience of being involved, of being present and participating in the clinical milieu to which the "case of Mrs. Jackson" refers.

Haunting aspects

Even if there were a library filled with books and articles about clinical responsibility, it would not have altered my experience that Saturday afternoon as I listened to the administrator on call describe Mrs. Jackson's turn of events. I was flooded with self-doubt and questions that I already knew could not be fully answered or settled. I thus found myself deep in the throes of a genuine *moral* experience, the kind, I knew, that often prompted my nursing and physician colleagues to request ethics consultation.

In that moment my practice of ethics consultation was transformed because *I* was transformed. No mere role-directed, institutionally legitimated actor, I now found myself squarely "inside" that which clinical ethics often addresses, "inside" in a manner that was deeply substantive. I too was experiencing what it was like to have an ethical stake in this situation because my actions had played, and would continue to play, a significant role in what was to be held as "good," "right," or "fair." After all, the administrator on call hoped I could confirm that she had "done the right thing."

But how could I, when I too was experiencing a sort of disbelief, an uncomfortability, and a disruptiveness in the now genuine link between Mrs. Jackson's broken jaw and her death. And in that moment of clarification, of wondering whether I could confirm that the administrator on call had "done the right thing," I saw that this would come down to a judgment – my judgment – about what I trusted, what

I believed, what I would be willing to live with in the aftermath of what came to be the decision. I too would become part of the decision-making nexus, the bearer of responsibility.

Uncertainty and change are hallmarks of clinical contexts and practice, including clinical ethics practice.[5] Mrs. Jackson's case is, in many ways, no different from every other ethics consultation in which I have been involved. All contain elements that, in hindsight – even of a few hours or the next day – point toward, to play on the title of one of Hans Jonas' final essays, "the burden and blessing of *morality*"[3]: Responsibility in practice often leaves one unsettled, uncertain, and face to face with one's own limitations.

Outcome

Many years have passed since this situation occurred. Since that time, I have been involved in more ethics consultations than I can remember without going through my files. Surprisingly, I remember most my conversation with Dr. McCord. It may be because he, who had not spent as much time with Mrs. Jackson or her daughter as had the nurses, was apparently more on the mark regarding Mrs. Jackson's best interests: she was more fragile than she appeared and most likely would have lingered and experienced the slow death he mentioned in his conversation with me. Thus, although he was more distant and detached from the patient than the nurses – they were, after all, spending 12 hours at a time with her (and her daughter) – Dr. McCord seemed to "see" Mrs. Jackson's interests more clearly.

Also of likely import is that I know from my own experience as well as from previous encounters with Gregg McCord that this was not intentional. He does not pay attention to subtleties of how patients, families, and nurses understand their situations and what they think is valuable. He even has acknowledged that part of what influenced his decision to become a surgeon was that he is "just not very good with people." He prefers the technical and procedural elements associated with surgery.

Over time I have trusted his assessment of himself and mine of him given our shared experience in other cases. Yet I cannot shake what I saw with Mrs. Jackson, a woman who died as a result of a broken jaw. I am reminded that just as much as I trust, I may be mistaken. And so, in yet another way, uncertainty about my own judgments and responsibility remains. And with that, I tread even more carefully whenever I am requested for ethics consultation.

Discussion questions

1. What responsibility do ethics consultants have for the outcome of cases on which they consult?

2. How should ethics consultants address, confront, and engage their own moral experiences?
3. How should the ethics consultant's moral experience factor into the recommendations she or he makes in a specific case?

REFERENCES

1. Zaner RM. Voices and time: The venture of clinical ethics. *J Med Philos*, 1993; 18(1): 9–31.
2. Bliton MJ, Finder SG. Traversing boundaries: Clinical ethics, moral experience, and the withdrawal of life supports. *Theor Med*, 2002; 23(3): 233–58.
3. Howe EG. Ethics consultants: Could they do better? *J Clin Ethics*, 1999; 10(1): 13–25.
4. Zaner RM. Listening or telling? Thoughts on responsibility in clinical ethics consultation. *Theor Med*, 1996; 17(3): 255–77.
5. Bliton MJ, Finder SG. The eclipse of the individual in policy (Where is the place for justice?). *Camb Q Healthc Ethics*, 1996; 5(4): 519–32.

Part V

The unspeakable/unassailable: religious and cultural beliefs

17

Adolescent pregnancy, confidentiality, and culture

Donald Brunnquell

Case narrative

Bena is a 14-year-old girl who is a member of a small, extremely close-knit immigrant community. She came to the emergency department with severe abdominal pain on a Tuesday night. She has been raised in the United States, speaks English as a primary language in school, and seems completely acculturated, but her mother and extended family immigrated shortly before she was born. Her mother does not speak English, and an interpreter is required for any discussions with staff. Bena lives with her mother and four siblings, but her mother was not available because she was working.

Bena said her pain had been going on for two days, and she initially denied sexual activity. When her urine pregnancy test came back positive, she admitted she had been sexually active with a cousin about her age. Further evaluation revealed an ectopic pregnancy. She was admitted to the hospital for further evaluation and treatment including consultation with an ob-gyn. Because this was a pregnancy-related issue, she could by state law consent to treatment on her own. Child Protective Services was consulted but did not open a case since this was apparently consensual relations with a same-age peer. Bena called home and left a message for her mother that she was in the hospital and that her mother should call as soon as possible.

Bena talked with the social worker and physician in the emergency department and requested that they not tell her mother that she was pregnant or sexually active. She stated that her mother would not be able to keep this information from Bena's aunt and that the entire community would soon know that she is pregnant. If this were to happen her family would be disgraced and she would be an outcast and considered unmarriageable in the community. The social worker and the physician urged her to change her mind and allow them to inform her mother, but she remained adamant that this would mean irreparable harm to her reputation at home, in school, and in her community.

When her mother came to the hospital the next morning, she was told through an interpreter (who had agreed to total confidentiality for Bena) that Bena was having severe abdominal pain and that the team was continuing to assess what they should do. This was true to the extent that a consultation was being obtained, but it did not reveal Bena's ectopic pregnancy.

An ethics consultation was requested regarding withholding information from the mother and the risks of medical treatment unsupervised by a parent weighed against the social risks Bena described. Given the issue's immediacy, I acted as an individual consultant to the team and then discussed the case with other committee members to assure a wider perspective.

Over the next 24 hours it was determined that this pregnancy was in a fallopian tube, and a plan was developed to have Bena stay in the hospital for treatment with a single dose of methotrexate, a recognized therapy for ectopic pregnancy and the only treatment that avoids surgery. Methotrexate is best known for its use in chemotherapy, and while it is 80–90% effective for treating ectopic pregnancy, it also carries significant risks for the woman, including nausea, stomatitis, bone-marrow suppression, pneumonitis, elevated liver enzymes, and possible rupture of the fallopian tube. This treatment requires a follow-up after two weeks to assure that the treatment is successful and to assure there are no side effects and continued follow-up for about six weeks. The physicians involved and the literature emphasize strict compliance with the follow-up.

Issues addressed in the ethics consultation included whether to accept the consent of a minor even if legally permissible, whether the mother had an absolute right to know the full situation, whether Bena could be trusted to complete adequate medical follow-up, and how the social risks to Bena's future weighed against medical risks of the treatment. As a result of the consult, and with Bena's permission, a staff member from a women's advocacy group for Bena's community was consulted. The advocate confirmed that Bena's social fears were realistic and urged the staff not to share information about the pregnancy with Bena's mother or any other family member.

With the ethics consultant's agreement, the mother was not informed of the specific treatment being given or the reason for the treatment, was told that her daughter was receiving medication for pain, and was told that Bena would need to return for regular follow-up. The mother angrily questioned whether she was being told the truth but never requested to review the medical record. Bena was told that if she did not make all her follow-up appointments (daily for one week, then every other day for a week, then weekly for four weeks) the police would escort her to the appointment. Given the treatment's medical risks and the fact that she would not have adult supervision, this plan reflected the staff's insistence that follow-up be absolutely essential and nonnegotiable. While this was to some extent a threat, it was necessary to assure compliance if Bena did not adhere to the follow-up. Making her aware of the plan informed her of steps that would be taken, respecting her autonomy and emphasizing the importance of follow-up.

Professional reflections

Adolescent consent and autonomy issues have been frequently discussed.[1,2,3] Yet every dilemma involving adolescent autonomy in decision making and control of information is unique. The nature of the clinical situation, the nature of the decision, the capacity (as distinguished from legal competence) of the adolescent, the particulars of legal guardianship and family systems, the hospital ethos about decision making, and the social/cultural milieu all contribute to a final decision about whether and how to respect adolescent decision making and confidentiality. In this instance providers agreed on the recommended course of treatment, although other decisions were possible. A parent, for example, may have requested surgery, and that approach would have been honored because it is within the standard of care.

The major decision regarding autonomy in this case was informational. The team proceeded on the understanding that if persons are legally entitled to consent to their own treatment, they also are legally entitled to control the information about that treatment. The particular state law in question (Minnesota Statute 144.341–347)[4] does not resolve the ethical dilemma, however, because it holds that a provider *may* provide treatment on the consent of a minor in certain situations, not that a provider *must* act on the minor's consent. Careful evaluation of all the factors listed above becomes essential. In this instance the team concluded that Bena understood the risks and consequences of the proposed treatment and the alternatives.

More importantly, the team concluded that Bena's understanding of her family and community situation was reliable and should be accepted. There was no specific reason to disbelieve her; her account seemed plausible based on the provider's knowledge of the culture and the advocate's confirmation of that understanding. Yet the risk of the treatment argued that she should not be left totally alone in pursuing treatment. She produced no viable family adult who could be trusted. The result was a compromise of frequent direct medical follow-up with a clear consequence for not complying with follow-up. To everyone's relief, this plan was never needed, but the question remains: Is this threat of coercion an unwarranted diminution of her autonomy or a reasonable compromise that promotes autonomy with some oversight?

Haunting aspects

This case remains a troubling episode in attempting to balance truth-telling, adolescent autonomy, the weight of social and medical issues in evaluating risk, and the role of culture in deciding on the best course of treatment. Especially haunting were aspects of the unknown that came alive in this case. Was Bena's report of how she became pregnant accurate, and would she be adequately protected in the future? Was her estimate of the cultural impact of pregnancy on her future social role believable? What is the reality of her relationship with her mother, and could her mother in fact not keep information about her daughter confidential? Do these uncertainties justify withholding information from her mother as well as from any adult connected to Bena in her home community?

The uncertainties in this case weighed heavily on the staff members and me in light of the issue of not fully informing Bena's mother. This was not a matter of legal risk since legal advice regarding the state law held that Bena could give consent for pregnancy-related treatment. This was not a viable pregnancy, so it did not raise questions about abortion, a matter handled differently by the applicable state law.

Meeting with Bena's mother and repeatedly withholding information that she asked for was deeply disturbing to all involved, even if legal. While no "affirmative" lie was told, significant information was withheld. All involved felt this was tantamount to lying. In a medical environment that stresses family-centered care, and given a core belief that a 14-year-old should have a responsible adult involved in her life, the question of whether this was the best course of action haunted all the providers. The community advocate's affirmation reassured us that we had struck some kind of balance, but some providers questioned whether the advocate had "an agenda" with regard to emancipation and acculturation of women in the culture. The moral distress of this breach of the presumptive duty of truth-telling, albeit rationalized by nonmaleficence, lives with the providers to this day.

No one relaxed in the first week of treatment as questions about potential side effects and compliance with follow-up remained salient. There was some concern that Bena would "disappear" to another state with a large population from her community and be lost to follow-up. This was a calculated risk of not involving adults from her community. The threat of sending police to find her had the possibility of alienating her as well as the possibility of increasing compliance. This was, however, part of the compromise of not notifying an adult in her home community with whom she would have regular contact. Such threats are not typical for our practice, and they remain a source of discomfort in this case.

For the pregnancy of a 14-year-old, the issue of protection, and what actions should be taken to intervene in her environment troubled us all. Bena emerged from a culture where power remained largely with the males, a fact that cut both ways in our efforts to discern whether she would be safe. Given the privilege men typically hold in this culture, it seemed likely that Bena's single mother would be unable to adequately protect either her confidentiality or, in the future, her person. Lack of a true understanding of this family and culture made accurate assessment difficult and left lingering uncertainties about the decisions.

On further reflection, however, it is important to ask the degree to which we can know such factors even in familiar, "mainstream" culture. The wide variability of behavior across families assures us that at best our attempts to understand issues like protection and long-term social effects are guesswork. This does not, however, justify ignoring such issues and focusing on the purely medical risks of treatment.

The ethics consultation was carried out by a single consultant who used phone consultation with other members of the ethics committee for further review. These committee members analyzed the situation and decisions, but their responses were based on the information and description of the single consultant. This was driven by a practical need for repeated conversations with many members of the staff over a period of days. As the nexus of communication about the moral issues, this in itself felt burdensome. While the other committee members or team members could request to alter the type of ethics consultation being provided, major control over how the consultation proceeded remained with the individual consultant.

Yet the clinical situation did not allow days, or even hours, to pull together a more formal small-group consultation. Staff members were already speaking to the mother at the time of the initial ethics consultation – they needed to be advised about what they would discuss. The physicians were not on the unit when the advocate was present and relied on the ethics consultant and social worker for evaluation of the advocate's input. Delaying treatment (medical or surgical) for the ectopic pregnancy was risky, and with so many people involved communication of many viewpoints was difficult. This all feels like a burden, but it's the proper burden for an ethics consultant to bear.

In the end, caring for the "whole child" in the context of family and culture must remain our goal. The unknowns and risks we face in this endeavor are just part of the task. We are accustomed to working with the uncertainties of medicine. Medical treatment in this case is estimated to be 80–90% effective. The effectiveness of our decision not to inform the parent, to allow Bena to be the primary manager of her own care, and to trust her return for follow-up is unknown. Yet we must make judgments about these areas and live with the possibility that we make errors in judgment in spite of our best efforts. The possibilities of such errors do not fade from our memory.

Outcome

Bena was discharged from the hospital five days after she appeared at the emergency department and three days after she received the single dose of methotrexate. She tolerated the treatment well, the ectopic pregnancy was resolved, and she complied with her follow-up appointments. Bena's mother never learned of the pregnancy or the treatment. Bena maintained contact with the community advocate briefly after her final visits. She did not maintain contact to receive regular birth control.

Discussion questions

1. Do you believe withholding specific information from Bena's mother was lying? If so, was it justified?
2. Is there a minimum age at which a minor patient can be trusted, including their representations of sexual activity, their home situation, and their culture?
3. How should healthcare providers estimate the risks to a patient living in a cultural group that remains relatively isolated, with which the providers do not share a language, and to which the providers have little access to the real ethos of the cultural group?
4. Is it justifiable to raise the issue of police involvement to locate her if she does not comply with treatment, or is such a threat disrespectful or harmful?
5. How should this information have been documented in the medical chart, knowing that parents could request the chart?

REFERENCES

1. Gaylin W, Macklin R. *Who Speaks for the Child.* New York: Plenum Press, 1982.
2. Blustein J, Levine C, Dubler NN, eds. *The Adolescent Alone: Decision Making in Health Care in the United States.* New York: Cambridge University Press, 1999.
3. Alderson P, Sutcliffe K, Curtis K. Children's competence to consent to medical treatment. *Hastings Cent Rep*, 2006; 36(6): 25–34.
4. Minnesota Statute 144.241–347. State of Minnesota. Available at http://ros.leg.mn/bin/getpub.php?pubtype=STAT`CHAP`SEC&year=2006&section=144.341

18

"Tanya, the one with Jonathan's kidney": a living unrelated donor case of church associates

Tarris D. Rosell

Case narrative

An ethics consult was requested of me in my role as a fellow in transplantation ethics. It came from the kidney-transplant coordinator in regard to a potential living unrelated donor (LURD). Apparently the donor had minimal knowledge of and relationship to her intended recipient.

The case first came up for consideration in the transplant team's weekly meeting early in January. Transplant coordinator Callie Jenkins, RN, presented Tanya Keller's case following Ms. Keller's donor evaluation a few days earlier. The case required ethics input because of the potential donor's relational status to Jonathan Noble, the intended recipient with end-stage renal disease. Ms. Keller was said to be a "church associate" of Mr. Noble.

"What are our criteria for living donor acceptance?" asked a senior nephrologist, with a nod to the ethicist in attendance. "Uncoerced, not paid, understands the procedure, good health." The physician had answered his own question.

Shortly afterward, the transplant coordinator sent me a letter formally requesting an ethics consult:

Ms. Tanya Keller is a 31-year-old woman who has expressed a wish to donate a kidney to one of our patients, Jonathan Noble. She has been tissue typed and found to be a compatible match to Jonathan. Tanya describes herself as a church acquaintance/friend of Jonathan's. They have known each other awhile, though she does not describe their relationship as close.

Ms. Keller has not had the complete medical donor evaluation yet, but in our preliminary medical inquiry she sounds like a healthy candidate. Her reasons for wanting to donate seem sound. We have asked Tanya to see you to help her explore the full implication of kidney donation. This is part of our protocol for unrelated potential donors who do not have a "close" relationship with the recipient.

If you need any further information, please feel free to call me.

Thank you in advance for seeing this pleasant woman.

My initial consult note was drafted as a letter to the requestor. It included a summary of the facts as I understood them and the ethical issues this LURD case raised. The note was sent after several conversations with transplant clinicians, followed by telephone and face-to-face interviews conducted with the potential living donor:

In response to your request, I met with Ms. Tanya Keller for approximately one hour. As you had discovered also, Tanya is indeed a pleasant young woman who appears to have made her decision to be evaluated as a potential LURD from altruistic motivations that are in keeping with her commitments as a devout Pentecostal Christian.

Ms. Keller presents as a rather self-assured and professional young adult, competent, intelligent, and compassionate. In our session together, Tanya seemed quite able and willing to explore ethical and other concerns relevant to her donation decision, which she sees as having been that of agreeing to undergo the evaluation process with intent to follow through to surgery if the transplant team deems appropriate. She firmly believes that donation to Mr. Noble is an idea implanted in her mind by God.

This initially occurred during a Thanksgiving service at church, and Tanya believes that her assent is in cooperation with divine will. Knowledge of Jonathan Noble's medical situation came via their pastor's announcements from the pulpit and requests for prayer on Jonathan's behalf. Tanya claims that no one asked for donation, that she never before had entertained such a thought, that she does not know anyone who donated an organ, and that she had not seen the recent news documentary on LURD between church associates. All of this reaffirms in her mind the notion that this is "of God, not me."

According to Tanya, when she first approached the potential recipient, he expressed skeptical hesitation ("I would never ask this of anyone!"). She wondered if Jonathan thought her to be "crazy." He agreed to evaluation, she says, given her sense that "this really is from God." Asked if Mr. Noble's family is in agreement, Ms. Keller says: "They're thrilled! His mom came up and gave me a big hug the other day." Others in the church have sought her out, inquiring if she's "Tanya, the one with Jonathan's kidney?"

When I noted that this notoriety and recognition may also make it more difficult subsequently to say no to kidney donation, Tanya agreed but did not anticipate changing her decision.

Asked about support persons available during her anticipated recovery period, Ms. Keller says the church people "are very loving and caring," that she has friends from work also, and that "actually, Jonathan's mom is going to help out afterwards." She neither expects nor wants her own family around for assistance.

Ms. Keller is single (divorced) and believes that Mr. Noble is about her own age and single also. She admits, when asked, to possible romantic aspirations motivating her volunteerism, but she dismisses them on the basis that "the idea came so clearly from God and not from me."

However, her expectation of their relationship after the transplant is that "there would be some bonding, some special relationship." My suggestion that there could be avoidance of the donor by the recipient (due to feelings of obligation, guilt, etc.) was received thoughtfully. "Jonathan did say something about how he could never repay this, but I told him I didn't expect to be paid in any way." This posttransplant recipient-response uncertainty does not seem to deter her willingness to donate.

Ms. Keller is somewhat apprehensive about surgery but dismisses risks associated with donor nephrectomy: impact on future pregnancy, surgical mortality or morbidity, and potential poor outcomes. She also has a family history of diabetes but views whatever happens as "the will of God." This perspective and her commitments are buttressed by the expressed support of her pastor.

I spoke with Jonathan Noble in subsequent weeks. The first appointment occurred in my office immediately after Jonathan had endured a painfully botched attempt at hemodialysis. With toxins still accumulating in his undialyzed vascular system and the nerve-damaged arm throbbing, our initial conversation was cut short. During two subsequent occasions, Jonathan's account correlated with Tanya's in nearly all respects.

Jonathan was not eager for a close relationship with his donor posttransplant. While he appreciated her offer and was willing to accept a kidney on the premise that the idea ultimately was "of God," as Tanya claimed, Jonathan wanted her to know there was nothing he could give in return.

Tanya continued to assure all of us that her gift would be free and clear. At the same time, she anticipated "some bonding or special relationship" to result from this unusual sharing of a significant body part with someone who was both a "church associate" and virtually a stranger.

Professional reflections

In my ethics consultation note to Nurse Callie Jenkins, I referenced the apparent altruism, reinforced by religious norms, of the potential living unrelated kidney donor. Ethical concerns for informed consent were appropriately raised in this situation, due especially to (a) Tanya's lack of a prior relationship with the intended recipient, (b) her lack of clarity regarding motivations to donate and idealized expectations of a posttransplant relationship with the recipient, (c) some potentially coercive influences within the religious community of which Jonathan and his parents were long-term members but which Tanya had joined only recently – influences that (if present) could make a donor's decision insufficiently autonomous and freely chosen.

I believe that Ms. Keller was open and candid about her deliberations leading to donor evaluation. She also exhibited a willingness and capability to gain further insight into areas of her self-understanding impinging on this decision. "What is worrisome," I wrote, "is that Tanya's account of her decisional process gives evidence of loneliness being attenuated by submission to bodily harms."

The consult note concludes with a recommended course of action based on ethics concerns and worries. "Therefore, my recommendation would be to put off any LURD decision, strongly encouraging the potential donor to explore further these issues in short-term insight-oriented counseling. This should be followed by at least one additional conversation here regarding Ms. Keller's decisional status."

To leave the donation decision truly open and uncoerced, I urged that any consequent surgery be scheduled only after sustained counseling had occurred and after a conversation confirming consent had taken place.

Haunting aspects

The most obvious ethical challenge to living organ donation is the norm of *primum non nocere*: "first, do no harm." Donor nephrectomy seems a blatant violation of the ancient medical prohibition against surgically harming a patient for whom no physical benefit derives. The term "donor mutilation" was common parlance in the moral philosophy of some theological ethicists who pondered the permissibility of living organ donation in its early days.[1] I am personally haunted by the possibility that wrongful mutilation via donation occurred in this case, that Tanya Keller indeed may have had her "loneliness . . . attenuated by submission to bodily harms."

The ethical tension between harms and benefits explains our emphasis on donor-informed consent: "Uncoerced, not paid, understands the procedure, good health." But is that sufficient for living donation of a significant body part? Does anyone ever fully understand a procedure that is inherently a one-time experience? Can we ever get fully informed consent for a LURD nephrectomy?

If the living donor and recipient have a prior close relationship, transplant clinicians might justify donor harms by referencing the psychological benefits of saving a loved one from dialysis or early death. Clearly, even in this case of an unrelated donor – virtually a stranger to the intended recipient – some psychological and especially spiritual benefits were realized prior to surgery. There was a sense of adherence to altruistic Christian norms, the *agape* love required of the faithful on behalf of a sibling in faith. Relational benefit occurred as a matter of her enhanced role within the church family, regardless of whether a "special relationship" with Jonathan was to develop. There is much about this living organ donation that seems just right. Could it be otherwise?

Yet, something about the situation unsettles me. In part, I am troubled by the repeated references to this bodily donation (mutilation?) as "the will of God." Tanya insists that her donor inclination is "of God, not me." Is it so? Does God really ask, perhaps require, such a thing of lonely individuals? Christians quote a biblical injunction to "offer your bodies as living sacrifices, holy and pleasing to God – this is your spiritual act of worship."[2] The first-century writer could not have had living donation of a kidney in mind, but might a LURD be the epitome of modern-day application of an ancient principle? Or have we taken this altogether too far in our attempts to prolong life and forestall death? I am torn. There is for me a brewing conflict between the good accomplished by self-sacrificial donors emulating Jesus and the haunting suspicion that our willingness to accept (or even encourage) organic self-sacrifice is not all good.

"I thought too that Tanya seemed maybe kinda lonely," Nurse Callie Jenkins admitted upon reading my consult note regarding her potential LURD patient. Surely one way to deal with relational isolation is to become a part of a religious group. I am a Christian clergyman and a strong advocate of church affiliation. We speak metaphorically of church as a body with many members joined together. But becoming a part of the church body ought not to entail the loss of a body part. Even male genital circumcision, an ancient Jewish custom, became optional for Christian converts from the start of the Judeo-Christian Church. Have we now, in Tanya's case, religiously and tragically confused symbol and function, made literal the figurative?

In my consultation note, I suggested to Nurse Callie that her donor patient's "theology ought not to become the focus for further inquiry." In retrospect, given a second opportunity, I would ask a lot of theological questions. What *is* "the will of God" and what does this mean in the context of human ingenuity in biomedicine? Does God require of us everything that technologically *can* be done in the cause of life extension? Surely not; but what then is required of the faithful? Should Christian ministers use the biblical metaphors "body of Christ" and "spiritual family" if doing so becomes dangerous to the health of some "family" members who provide potential health benefits to others?

It is not coincidental that the living donor is female and her intended recipient is male. At the time of Tanya's offer, and every year since, the odds of this gender pairing in the United States are nearly 60/40. More women give up body parts and more men receive them.[3] "Tanya, the one with *Jonathan's* kidney?" Really? What's going on here? I am left to wonder – and to ponder my role as a relatively impotent ethics consultant still conflicted by the outcome.

Outcome

Follow-up conversations with Nurse Callie occurred after those with Tanya and Jonathan. Their transplant coordinator seemed to be stymied by the counseling recommendation I had made because it was unprecedented. Callie still appeared uncomfortable with the idea but agreed to proceed when we discussed my worries about "loneliness being attenuated by submission to bodily harms."

I discovered some weeks later that the nurse ultimately chose not to follow through with the plan. Why not? Perhaps because the psychiatry consultant was more comfortable than I was with moving forward. Perhaps because an international shortage of donor kidneys ensures that momentum is always toward accepting any healthy organ that comes along. In addition, Nurse Callie resigned from the transplant center midway through the donor-evaluation process. The case was transferred temporarily to another overloaded transplant coordinator who passed it to Callie's eventual replacement shortly before already-scheduled donor and transplant surgeries in early summer.

Noting that nothing had been done with regard to counseling follow-up, the new transplant coordinator, Jane, asked if I would contact the scheduled donor and recipient to assess their current state of willingness to proceed.

Jonathan was upbeat about the impending transplant and volunteered additional information on his relationship with Tanya. While expressing appreciation for her donor intent and also liking Tanya as a new church friend and someone who "seems like a nice person," Jonathan also stated that he had been clear with his donor-to-be that no "special relationship" should be expected afterward. "And she seemed OK with that."

It turns out that Tanya had been introduced to a living donor kidney recipient doing well ten years post-transplant. Tanya was of course interested in the living donor's status. She reported her findings to me with evident concern: "He had a big incision and they punctured his lung, so he had a lot of pain. But I don't think that will happen to me. They're supposed to use a smaller incision nowadays."

"Yet there are those risks," I reflected. "You can always say, 'No.'" Tanya told me she had no intention of backing out at this point.

There was one thing Tanya failed to mention to me. The medical center's public relations department had contacted Jane to tell her that a local television station was following the Keller-Noble case. How had the media become involved? Jane did not know. Did Jonathan or his family call the television station or was it possibly Tanya herself? Might some other church associate – perhaps even the pastor – have considered this a good story for public relations or for "the glory of God"?

More likely, media involvement came at the request of someone within the transplant program and medical center intending to raise organ-donor awareness along with the institution's public image. Sensing a heartwarming human-interest story with religious overtones, a television journalist had already interviewed Tanya and Jonathan and had filmed them in church and elsewhere. Jane expressed hesitation about this turn of events. "I told them this is my first case; I hope they don't interview me. The media coverage could be wonderful for donation, but I sure hope everything goes well. I just hope everything turns out alright."

Two days later, with television cameras rolling, both surgeries proceeded according to plan. Postoperative clinical reports indicated that both the recipient and the donor were doing well.

Discussion questions

1. Ethicists might call what Tanya did for Jonathan a "supererogatory" act, one that goes over and above what is required or expected of persons. Could that ever be wrong?
2. Given the ever-widening gap between the supply of donor kidneys and those who could benefit from them, should clergy persons encourage and

solicit among their congregation living organ donation to prolong the life of another?

3. What should be the role of an ethics consultant in situations when the "ought" or "ought not" seems to be going in a direction opposite to the consultant's own moral judgments? Is consultation a morally neutral role or should ethicists be moralists sometimes?

4. Can media coverage of a medical story create undue influence on patient and medical team decision making?

REFERENCES

1. Cunningham B. The morality of organic transplantation. In: *Studies in Sacred Theology*, No. 86. Washington, DC: Catholic University of America Press; 1944. To my knowledge, this doctoral dissertation is the first book-length treatise on the ethics of living donor issues. Reverend Cunningham, a Catholic priest, was interested primarily in ovary transplants.

2. *Romans 12:1*. New International Version of the New Testament.

3. The Organ Procurement and Transplantation Network. Available at http://www.optn.org

19

Futility, Islam, and death

Kathryn L. Weise

Case narrative

Some cases stay with us because communication goes awry despite our best efforts, because hoped-for outcomes elude us, or because we make bonds with patients or families in deep or unexpected ways. In the aftermath of this case, I felt shaken to the core, questioning my role as a physician-ethicist. It drove home a profound respect for the strain we escalate by asking families to confront death head-on.

For several weeks during biweekly multidisciplinary rounds in the medical intensive-care unit (ICU), the staff updated the bioethicist on-call about Sharma, a 24-year-old woman with acute myelogenous leukemia who had suffered cardiac arrest on the oncology ward after beginning chemotherapy. She had been resuscitated but remained comatose from severe, irreversible brain damage. Looking at her lying inert in bed was wrenching even to me as a seasoned intensivist. She was massively swollen and bruised, festooned with IV lines, support machines, and tubes, and oozing blood from almost every line site and bandage, epitomizing "invasive" and "aggressive" therapy. Her nurses and doctors looked sobered and almost angry, but they were quiet and gentle at her bedside. Her leukemia was still active, but she could not receive further chemotherapy because of her multiple organ system damage.

All physicians and nurses involved in her care now believed that comfort care rather than intensive care was the only medically appropriate thing to do since her underlying leukemia could not be treated. Her mother and durable power of attorney for health care, Mrs. Abu, refused to allow withdrawal of support based on her religious beliefs. A bioethics consult was requested to help mediate further discussions with the patient's family. The ICU team had met with Mrs. Abu on numerous occasions before asking for the consult and had involved an imam to help the family reach decisions consistent with the patient's Islamic faith. The staff conveyed to the consultant a sense of moral outrage at being asked to provide what they felt was cruel rather than kind care.

In our ethics consultation process, an individual consultant usually begins a consult and may complete it if the issue is straightforward and if a mutually acceptable resolution can be reached without involving other ethicists. There is a mechanism for using a small-group approach in cases that involve potential unilateral decision making by the medical team against the wishes of the patient or family. In this case, the individual consultant reached an impasse and called for a small-group committee consult when the medical team began asking about discontinuing support against the mother's wishes because of medical futility. My involvement began as a member of the hospital ethics committee and member of the small-group consult team. I gathered background information from the medical staff, the medical record, and the original bioethics consult. Sharma's leukemia had not responded to alternative medicine approaches in her home state so she had entered a hospice setting there and agreed to a do-not-resuscitate (DNR) order. An older sister had died one year earlier of leukemia after alternative medicine approaches failed. She had been admitted to our oncology ward for a second opinion after her father, who did not follow the same faith and was estranged from her mother, persuaded her to obtain a second opinion. She consented to undergo chemotherapy. No DNR order was written, which later became a source of great anger and distrust among her family members. In our hospital, it is customary to honor outside DNR orders in the emergency room setting, but they must be rewritten on hospital forms to ensure that patients' most recent wishes are being honored. Her oncologist's note in the medical record stated that the patient and both parents understood that her chances of treatment-related mortality would be high and chances of success were low, and each expressed a willingness to proceed with aggressive therapy, "thus removing her from hospice and a supportive-care-only approach despite these risks." Mrs. Abu did not recall being present for any discussions about resuscitation status and felt that her daughter was only in her current unwanted situation because an order had not been written prior to the arrest. Her faith interpretation dictated that once an intervention starts it must continue because only Allah can determine when a person will die.

After extensive discussion with Sharma's medical-care team, the small-group committee supported the assessment of medical futility but stressed that this opinion did not obligate the medical team to discontinue support against family wishes. We recommended that if unilateral discontinuation of support were to be pursued, the family should be given at least 48 hours notice so it could make other arrangements, seek legal recourse, or come to terms with the decision. I offered to meet with Sharma's mother, the ICU attending physician, and another member of the small-group consult team. The ICU attending chose to participate in that meeting rather than unilaterally discontinue support. Mrs. Abu, the patient's surviving sisters, a large extended family, and the social worker involved in the case were also present. Sharma's father declined to attend. Family members were furious with the hospital staff because a DNR order had not been written, which made it difficult to progress beyond repeated demands to explain why. Another meeting was arranged with the family, the oncologist who the family saw as failing to write the DNR order, and myself, but the family's anger was not diminished by the oncologist's agreement that in retrospect he also had regrets. Her family steadfastly refused to limit support in the ICU and asked that we arrange transfer back to her home state. Over the course of the next week, the social worker and I investigated ways to achieve this request, but it proved impossible because of her medical instability, inability to find a facility out of state that would accept her on a ventilator for hospice care, and costs to the family and the institution.

I arranged and attended several other family meetings. During the first of these, the ICU attending physician again reviewed her medical status and presented the neurologists' opinion that she was unlikely to awaken. Mrs. Abu was not able to come to the next meeting because she felt ill. I spoke with her by telephone through a daughter, who asked us all to "back off" because her mother was having stomach pains and could not come to the telephone. At the next in-person meeting, it became clear that Mrs. Abu knew her daughter was dying, but she was firm in refusing discontinuation of support. We discussed goals and wishes at length, trying to agree on an approach to care that would honor Sharma's earlier beliefs, fit with her religion, and seem to her medical team as if the team were acting in a medically appropriate way.

It became increasingly difficult to participate in family meetings because it was painful to hear such anger, to see such pain, and to be unable to help abate it. It was painful to be part of a group being blamed. I faced each meeting with hope and left each one feeling deflated. I felt the pressure of time because Sharma seemed suspended in a horrible state, her family's anguish was being prolonged, and the staff was so clearly in moral pain. This was not a case in which endless patience or meeting after meeting seemed to help. The pressure from staff, pushing harder to end this distressing chapter, was intense.

Finally, Mrs. Abu agreed that if we could transfer Sharma to a local hospice setting she would allow hospice care, including removing her from the ventilator. I would like to think that we had finally shown that we cared, that we accepted rather than deflected her anger, and that we had made a good-faith effort to send her home, but I worry that instead we had only worn her down through our persistence. It seemed as if Mrs. Abu had abandoned her religious beliefs in the face of our repeated pleas to let Sharma die peacefully. Several days later Sharma was transferred to a local inpatient hospice on a ventilator, blood pressure support, and pain medications. A palliative-care physician had accepted her in spite of mechanical ventilation and blood pressure support with agreement from her family to shift to comfort care within 24 hours of admission. Sharma arrived safely at hospice, remained ventilated and on pressor support overnight, and then died after extubation the next morning with multiple family members at her side.

Later that day I learned that Mrs. Abu had suffered a massive heart attack and died several hours before the death of her daughter.

Haunting aspects

As the consultant, I was stunned. I knew that we had not caused her heart disease, but I felt that by failing to recognize that Mrs. Abu's illness was serious, an element of caring for this family was missed. I had been proud that we, the ethics consultation service and hospital, had done the best we could under the circumstances. We found a compromise that would allow Sharma's death to occur in a place that Mrs. Abu accepted. What about this sudden, unexpected death was so difficult to accept? I am a pediatric intensive-care physician with more than 20 years of experience in that field. In that role, one of my skills is anticipating problems to avoid complications or further deterioration in my patients. I mentally and emotionally share responsibility for what happens to my patients even when they are not solely in my care. Also, as a pediatrician, I see a patient's family as being integral to the illness and recovery process.

What ran through my head when I learned of Mrs. Abu's death? The internal dialogue went something like this. I knew Mrs. Abu was sick, but her daughter told me it was a stomach problem, not that she had heart disease . . . [*but I didn't ask . . . it wasn't my business to ask . . . but I would have asked if this had been the mother of one of my patients . . . but what about her privacy? . . . she wouldn't have had to tell me, but I should have asked . . .*] But I was the bioethics consultant – I was not anybody's doctor . . . [*I am always a doctor . . .*] I do not practice adult medicine . . . [*Rationalization! I am still fundamentally a doctor.*] The patient in the adult ICU was not my patient in the same way that children in the pediatric ICU are my patients. Would knowing that she was ill have changed what I tried to arrange in this case from an ethics perspective? [*No.*] Would it have changed how I worked on this case? [*Maybe.*] Was I ever unkind to them? [*No, at least it didn't feel like it at the time.*] I knew this was stressful to everyone, including me . . . but was it my job to understand just how stressful? [*Yes, but not my job alone.*] Would Mrs. Abu have sought medical help if I had suspected a serious illness and offered help? [*Probably only alternative therapies, given the past choices her daughters made, but I shouldn't make that assumption – and maybe those therapies would have helped her.*] Did I become blind to the needs of Mrs. Abu in this process because I was working under a mission to discontinue intensive care on this patient? [*Maybe.*] Will this change what I do during future bioethics consultations? [*Yes, I will be more aware of the stress that bioethicists foster – because we sometimes orchestrate focus on the most stressful issues in life.*]

This case haunted me because I felt that I did a good job as the bioethicist but missed something very important to my identity as a physician-ethicist. It made me realize in a very deep way that while we sometimes decrease or diminish stress for families by clarifying issues and by spending time with them, at other times we drill down to those issues in ways that may heighten the pain of those who will survive.

Professional reflections

I am often aware of role boundaries while doing ethics consultations, but this case brought them more clearly to the forefront than other cases. When consulting on an ethical issue at bedside, I am sorely tempted to ask physicians in training if they recognize the respiratory distress of the patient in front of us. I will usually find a way to do that, remembering that this is not my patient but knowing also that this young physician truly may not see what I am seeing. In the process, I try to remember that if I am perceived as meddling where I am not wanted or seen as stepping out of the role of ethicist, the medical team may be less likely to ask for an ethics consult on other patients. I also know that in those interactions I am acting as a physician-educator, not as an ethicist. This is a shift from one role to another rather than confusion over role boundaries.

Although in early clinical ethics literature some advocated for only clinicians to undertake ethics consultation,[1] more recently authors such as Agich have described an approach in which clinician or nonclinician ethics consultants are accepted as an equal part of the healthcare team. In this model, the basic task of the consultant is "to undertake a thorough investigation and analysis of a case and provide sound ethical advice through recommendations that respect the different viewpoints of the individuals involved in a case."[2] The emphasis is on understanding the medical aspects of the case enough to craft ethical recommendations that are in line with patient values and values of the medical team but not to make medical practice decisions. In Sharma's case, a medical judgment was initially made – agreement with the medical team's assessment that continuing aggressive interventions would not result in clinical improvement. The ethical recommendation evolved from that judgment. Perhaps the close relationship of those parts of the process, plus my own background as a managing physician in an ICU, helped blur my own professional boundaries.

As an intensivist, responsibility for orchestrating complex and sometimes disheartening situations is part of daily work. As an ethicist on this case, I orchestrated what I might have left to others more responsible for some aspects of her care, including a plan for discharge to a hospice setting. It has always been a challenge to balance keeping a clinical "distance" from patients and families during medical care against the need to recognize the emotional needs of families and of myself. I have often told myself that if I lose either the ability to stay emotionally even-keeled in intense situations or the ability to feel truly sad or happy, then it will be time to stop practicing medicine. In my mind and heart, the same applies to practicing ethics consultation. Sharma and Mrs. Abu reminded me of how difficult it is to separate roles that we play in parallel or simultaneously, even when we are called to play only one. We are fallible, and we learn from each chapter we help to write.

On a more formal note, as a consultant on this case I became more familiar with how certain Islamic teachings about end-of-life care impacted this case. African American Islamic beliefs surrounding death are guided by Middle Eastern and African Islamic interpretations of the Qur'an and by those parts of the Islamic Code of Medical Ethics that address the sanctity of human life.[3,4] Life is viewed as sacred, given to man by Allah and only to be taken away by Allah. It is stated in the Qur'an that " . . . if anyone slay a person – unless it be for murder or spreading mischief in the land – it would be as if he slew the whole people. And if anyone saved a life, it would be as if he saved the life of the whole people."[5] Allah is seen as the owner and giver of life, and his rights to give and take life are not to be violated by human beings,[6] which guides thought on suicide and euthanasia. The concept of a life "not worth living" does not exist in Islamic thought.

Islamic scholar Hassan Hathout interprets a portion of the Islamic Code of Medical Ethics by stating that "when treatment . . .carries no prospect of cure, it ceases to be mandatory . . . but no action should be taken to actively bring about death."[7] This would seem to guide physicians to show patience (a great virtue in Islam),[7] allowing death to occur on high levels of support rather than by actively withdrawing life-support measures in favor of comfort care. This creates a quandary for many Western physicians, whose interpretation of secular biomedical ethics may promote withdrawal of support in dying patients as a beneficent or nonmaleficent act. This conflict of perceived obligations – an Islamic family obeying sacred teachings by refusing to actively withdraw support, and Western physicians obeying guidance to do no harm through fruitless medical interventions – frequently causes an impasse.

Outcome

Physicians and other staff involved were informed of Sharma's death and were told about her mother's death. In discussion with various physicians, it became clearer that the admitting physicians assumed that because Sharma was opting for chemotherapy, a DNR order was no longer appropriate. We also discussed the role of clergy in such cases. While spiritual care can sometimes be helpful, in this case it could not resolve the quandary of whether to discontinue intensive therapies in a dying patient against family wishes. Our cooperative relationship with the local inpatient hospice was strengthened, though we all agreed that transferring a patient on intensive-care therapies to that setting should rarely be done. Multiple caregivers learned more about this family's interpretation of Islamic teachings. I remain haunted both by my inability to separate my roles as physician and ethicist and by the power we have as ethicists to help and to hurt. At the same time, I am comforted by recognizing that insight, though often painful, can lead to growth.

Discussion questions

1. Would this case have been better handled by a small- or large-group committee model than by a single-consultant model? Why?
2. Propose an approach to this case that would have been less stressful to family members and medical staff.
3. Discuss different formulations of futility as they apply to this case.
4. How important is it to maintain good relations with the medical team so that it will request the help of ethics consultation?
5. Do clinician-ethicists have a medical responsibility for family members when they are acting as ethics consultants? Could this divide their attention and perspective to the detriment of a good, focused ethics review?

REFERENCES

1. LaPuma J, Schiedermayer DL. The clinical ethicist at the bedside. *Theor Med*, 1991; 12: 141–9.
2. Agich GJ. Joining the team: Ethics consultation at the Cleveland Clinic. *HEC Forum*, 2003; 15(4): 310–22.
3. Islamic Code of Medical Ethics. *World Med J*, 1982; 29(5): 78–80.
4. *Islamic Code of Medical Ethics – the Sanctity of Human Life*. Available at http://www.islamset.com/ethics/code/sancti.html
5. Qur'an 5:32. Quoted in Hathout H. *Reading the Muslim Mind*. Plainfield, IN: American Trust Publications, 1995; 130.
6. Hathout H. *Reading the Muslim Mind*. Plainfield, IN: American Trust Publications, 1995; 131–5.
7. Hathout H. Islamic basis for biomedical ethics. In: Pellegrino E, Mazzarella P, Corsi P, eds. *Transcultural Dimensions in Medical Ethics*. Frederick, MD: University Publishing Group, Inc., 1992; 69.

20

Suffering as God's will

Kathrin Ohnsorge and Paul J. Ford

Case narrative

The clinical ethics consultation service received a telephone call from Dr. Cedar, an attending hospitalist. He briefly explained that Mr. Carnegie, a 70-year-old man, was refusing surgery for what Dr. Cedar described as a life-threatening bowel obstruction. The patient had been hospitalized repeatedly over the last 10 years for his underlying end-stage chronic obstructive pulmonary disease (COPD) with accompanying hypertension. He had periodically needed mechanical ventilation in the past and would likely need it again as his COPD worsened. According to Dr. Cedar, Mr. Carnegie had three viable treatment options: (a) undergo a relatively high-risk surgery to resolve the obstruction, (b) be discharged with total parenteral nutrition (TPN), suctioning, and a do-not-resuscitate (DNR) order, and (c) be discharged with palliative medicine/hospice care, a DNR order, and no means for feeding and hydration.

The patient was refusing surgery, refusing TPN, and refusing to have a DNR order written. He also refused to talk with the palliative medicine group. Dr. Cedar believed the patient was globally competent, but there were inconsistencies in the patient's decision making that called into question his capacity related to treatment options. Dr. Cedar noted that the patient had no more than a high school level of education. Dr. Cedar requested that the ethics consultants meet with him and the patient. He indicated that a decision needed to be made because "good medicine requires a consistent care plan." We went to the unit to meet face to face with the physician and patient.

In this case, the "we" of the ethics consultation service consists of a full-time clinical ethicist (PF) and a visiting bioethics doctoral candidate from Europe (KO). The ethics consultation service operates on a single-consultant model with an ethics committee backup in a 900-bed teaching/research hospital.[1] As part of the teaching mission of the institution, KO shadowed PF during a two-month internship.

On the unit we briefly met with the physician before talking with Mr. Carnegie. The patient's increased secretions made him difficult to understand. He believed his lung disease constituted his most serious illness and that there was nothing significantly wrong with his bowel. He said, "The doctors say I won't survive a surgery. Only God knows when it's my time. I've had plenty of surgeries and I am tired of them. I just don't want to be cut on no more." Mr. Carnegie did not fully appreciate the seriousness of his bowel obstruction, but he was well aware of the burdens of surgeries. He believed his life expectancy was approximately three to six months due to his lung disease. He had "lived a good life," felt ready to accept death, and believed that "God will guide" him and "direct" his course of treatment. He generally displayed coherent thinking. Mr. Carnegie asked us to return the following day to meet with his wife as well.

The next day, the patient, his wife, his two cousins, the physician in charge, and the bioethicist (PF) met at the bedside. The cousins reported that the doctors gave the patient a 20% chance of surviving a surgical intervention. However, in a meeting with the bioethicists beforehand, Dr. Cedar said Mr. Carnegie's surgical survival rate stood at approximately 90% but that he only had a 50% chance of surviving to be discharged from the hospital. During the family meeting, Dr. Cedar declined to offer percentages. He instead focused on the overall plan. He was confident that the patient would survive an operation. He spent nearly an hour explaining various treatment options. He continued to believe there were only three reasonable options. The family asked whether the patient could try eating by mouth. The physician agreed to try it but stated that there was less than a 5% chance of the obstruction resolving on its own. There was a high likelihood of the patient vomiting and aspirating because of the oral intake. The patient, who had been quiet during the whole discussion, agreed to go home on TPN, but he said he did not want to have a nasal gastric (NG) tube placed since this would make his throat sore. When the patient was asked why he would refuse surgery but still want to be resuscitated, he said: "CPR is what is generally done for all patients." He believed that everything was in God's hands and that God would decide whether he would live or die.

The bioethicist asked the patient about his religious beliefs since he had mentioned prayer and God several times. At that moment the physician, who had spent an hour in the meeting, excused himself to care for other patients. The expressions and "eye-rolling" of Mr. Carnegie and his family suggested they interpreted his departure as a disregard for God and spiritual questions.

Once invited to speak about spirituality, the patient and his family began to open up and become livelier. Mr. Carnegie expressed a strong nondenominational Protestant faith. In the last 25 years he had done only what God had wanted him to do. He knew God's will through direct communication, which he clarified as coming through influence on his actions and not through a voice. Mr. Carnegie explicitly said to the bioethicist, "God is working through these doctors and through you. You're here to help. But you know, sometimes doctors depend too much on themselves; then God does not work through them." Mr. Carnegie went on to say that his suffering must be for a purpose, and only God would know this purpose. In this vein, he declined all pain medications. He agreed to whatever God had planned for his life, and God would let him know about that plan. Throughout the conversation, he was calm and decisive. He seemed rather matter-of-fact, not at all fanatical. He explained his beliefs and values in coherent terms and provided consistent reasons for his beliefs. When asked if he wanted to speak with a hospital chaplain, Mr. Carnegie declined, saying that his cousin was a minister and that was enough. The bioethicist encouraged him, together with his family, to think about a decision overnight and "to ask God for an answer." This seemed a reasonable course since this was the way in which the patient routinely made decisions.

Professional reflections

There were a number of interesting lessons to be learned on a professional level. The first was a reminder about medical uncertainty. In this case, chart notes from the surgical team and the hospitalist both emphatically predicted that the patient would die without bowel surgery. This turned out to be wrong, since the bowel problem (probably an ileus rather than an obstruction) resolved on its own. The activities in ethics consultation were premised on misplaced medical certainty. Additionally, the case was presented as having only three "rational" solutions. As the clinical ethicists, we did not need to accept these as the only solutions. Perhaps the patient could have gone home on TPN without a written DNR order. There may have been a failure to fully explore reasonable alternatives by allowing the medical team to quickly define the parameters without further questioning.

Allowing the consult requester to define the ethics question may also have led to challenges. Dr. Cedar said the reason for the ethics consultation was the patient's inconsistent decision making. At first, this "ethical diagnosis" by the physician seemed appropriate: the fact that Mr. Carnegie refused the surgery but still wanted to be resuscitated seemed contradictory. Mr. Carnegie knew he had a life-limiting condition and did not want intrusive surgical interventions. Yet he also insisted on intrusive, and perhaps futile, resuscitative measures. However, to accept this as the ethical dilemma would have led to a closing off of other interpretations of the patient's decision making. Simply relying on the consult requester to define the ethical dilemma may lead a consultant to ignore alternate possibilities or additional complexities.

A further challenge for the clinical ethicists was the patient's unusual articulation of his decision-making process. He said his decisions were directed through a personal communication with God. In this case, should we have consulted a psychiatric service? After talking to the patient, we believed he had stated his beliefs in a clear, consistent manner. This was supported by his family's description of his values and decision-making processes. Mr. Carnegie's coherent decision making was backed by a personal set of beliefs. Given the family's support of the patient and the apparent consistency of wishes, we speculated that introducing a specialist from the psychiatric service would have disrupted the tenuous trust Mr. Carnegie held toward healthcare providers. No one who interacted with Mr. Carnegie claimed that he was delusional, delirious, or psychotic.

In a case like this, we interpret our professional responsibilities as hermeneutical: in order to uncover inconsistencies in the decision-making process we had to clarify the patient's underlying assumptions, preconceptions, and belief systems as well as those of his family, physicians, healthcare structures, and our own as bioethicists.[2,3] This is not a theoretical enterprise but rather one enacted through practical experience, communication, and deliberation.[4,5,6,7] In this sense, we reflected together with the patient, his family, and the physician on questions of the DNR order, the role of the patient's religious beliefs, and his being a member of a minority population. We also questioned the physician's inferences about the patient's capacity that appeared to be based largely on the patient's limited educational background. Finally, we considered the influences of our own spiritual beliefs. The foundational reasoning behind fears, preconceptions, and beliefs had to be understood and accounted for to support shared decision making.[8,9]

Haunting aspects

Did one author's (PF) use of religious language, given that he did not share the patient's faith tradition, mislead Mr. Carnegie into thinking the author was a believer? Did he manipulate the patient? At a minimum, there was the danger of appearing disingenuous. These were the risks of using the patient's language to validate the patient's way of understanding the world. Even if the patient's way of thinking of "God" was a psychological tool for his own mind, it appeared to be worth talking to him in his own language. But somehow this way of interacting seemed less than transparent. It felt deceptive as the words rolled off the author's tongue. Perhaps this was simply a tool to garner trust that otherwise would not have been gained if the patient knew the truth about the author's beliefs.

The influence of a collaborator/observer present during consultation must be recognized. The doctoral candidate (KO) in this case was very interested in issues of cultural differences. Having this trainee present could have influenced the primary consultant (PF) in a positive or negative way. After all, teachers want to instruct, but they also want to impress their students. Were there any compromises or missteps unintentionally made in the interest of making the primary consultant look compassionate or to punctuate a teaching point? In addition, we recognize that having more people present at a meeting naturally alters the group dynamics. In this way, just having an extra person in the room may have shifted the discussion.

As an observer, KO saw the challenges for bioethicists in similar cases as threefold: the dangers of entering the sphere of cultural/spiritual dialogue with little training in religious language, the dangers of imposing their own spiritual values on the patient, and the dangers of causing feelings of abandonment in the patient. Ethicists are seldom trained in religious issues or language. Using this language can lead to misunderstandings or misinterpretations without a good understanding of the context. Should ethicists strive, therefore, for basic training in religious issues or for counseling from a pastoral service? It is commendable that ethicists strive for additional training in religious issues so they can understand patients' needs in the most appropriate and professional way. And of course, professional handling of spiritual issues in bioethics cases requires close collaboration with other professionals in spiritual care as well as sensitivity for the limits of spiritual competence. Consulting a religious expert to answer questions for the consultant can provide important insights. In our case, we did not ask pastoral service for counseling because Mr. Carnegie did not want the pastoral service involved and because the patient's cousin was a minister who could support Mr. Carnegie. Some challenges for bioethicists in a case like this are no different from challenges seen with beliefs based on foundational nonreligious values. One can even imagine situations in which listening with a religiously untrained ear and with an open mind could give rise to fresh and new options. However, the richness of meaning in religious language may not always be apparent to those who have little training. Perhaps with more training we could have asked different questions that would have resulted in a clearer understanding.

Second, since all people necessarily hold spiritual or metaphysical beliefs (the absence of which would be a belief in itself), we as bioethicists naturally run the risk of unduly influencing patients by imposing our beliefs on them. A situation like the described case has great potential to generate a type of psychological countertransference: the way we project our own values and ideas toward patients or filter what we hear through our own metaphysical beliefs may distort our understanding of patients' beliefs and needs. Without constantly acknowledging and controlling for our own assumptions, we run the risk of manipulating patients into decisions they otherwise would not have made. Again, this is not a specific challenge of consultations with spiritual issues but of consultation in general. As in any counseling situation, bioethicists should constantly recognize their own beliefs and values as influencing factors in the consultation process. This is an underestimated challenge in ethics consultation.

Third, introducing God as a decision-maker could give the patient the impression that the bioethicist is avoiding offering helpful advice. The patient could feel more alone and abandoned than before because of this perceived shirking of duty. Part of the work in ethics consultation is helping patients recognize their values in a way that provides an integrated experience. In this case Mr. Carnegie explained his trust in God as his lifelong way of making decisions. There is a fine line between supporting a decision-making process and abandoning the patient by not providing guidance.

By encouraging Mr. Carnegie "to think about it overnight and to ask God for advice" we attempted to validate his way of being. The time frame in this medical situation made it possible to act in this way. However, in the absence of a response from the patient the next day, how long would we leave the question of therapy choice unanswered? We believe that at some point the bioethicist has a responsibility to help the patient make decisions in different ways when no decision comes forward. Fortunately the story went differently, and the delay, in fact, made clear the fallibility of the original medical judgment. But there are times when deferring to a patient's religious tradition to answer the question may just be a dodge by the ethicist assisting in difficult decision making.

Outcome

We came back the next afternoon. The patient said he had not heard from God so he had not made a decision. He continued to express faith that God would direct his course of treatment. When we returned the second day the patient was alert and smiling. He told us that the physicians believed his bowel problem had resolved. We met with Dr. Cedar. He said the patient appeared to be significantly better and did not need surgery. The patient was now eating solid food and was not vomiting. The patient was discharged to home the following day without a DNR order. He was also eating by mouth. Had his faith saved him? Or, did the pervasive uncertainty endemic to medical prognostication create a false picture? How could we tell the difference? Does it matter for the practice of bioethics? These questions certainly come to mind as we face other patients with beliefs different from our own.

Discussion questions

1. What are possible responses to a patient who selectively asserts that God is working through some members of the medical staff but not others?
2. Is failing to disclose a bioethicist's religious worldview deceptive if religious language is going to be used? In particular, is it deceptive or coercive if a clinical ethicist adopts language that does not reflect her particular worldview?
3. When, if ever, is it appropriate to suggest a psychiatric consult when a patient refers to a deity talking to them? Is that a sufficient condition?
4. The physicians were wrong about the terminal nature of the bowel obstruction. It resolved on its own. What influence, if any, should this lack of accuracy have on the way in which clinical ethicists address future cases with this particular set of physicians?

REFERENCES

1. Agich GJ. Joining the team: ethics consultation at the Cleveland Clinic. *HEC Forum*, 2003; 15(4): 310–22.
2. Dzur AW. Democratizing the hospital: deliberative-democratic bioethics. *J Health Polit Policy Law*, 2002; 27(2): 177–211.
3. Gadamer HG. *Wahrheit und Methode*. Tübingen: Mohr, 1960.
4. Grazia D. Moral deliberation: the role of methodologies in clinical ethics. *Med Health Care Philos*, 2001; 4: 223–32.
5. Habermas J. *Erläuterungen zur Diskursethik*. Frankfurt am Main: Suhrkamp, 1991.
6. Leder D. Toward a hermeneutical bioethics. In: Dubose E, Hamel R, O'Connell L, eds. *A Matter of Principles?* Valley Forge, PA: Trinity Press International, 1994; 240–59.
7. Ricoeur P. *Temps et récit, I*. Paris: Editions du Seuil, 1983.
8. Parker M. A conversational approach to ethics. In: Ashcroft R, Lucassen A, Parker M, Verkerk M, Widdershoven G, eds. *Case Analysis in Clinical Ethics*. Cambridge: Cambridge University Press, 2005; 149–64.
9. Widdershoven G. Interpretation and dialogue in hermeneutic ethics. In: Ashcroft R, Lucassen A, Parker M, Verkerk M, Widdershoven G, eds. *Case Analysis in Clinical Ethics*. Cambridge: Cambridge University Press, 2005; 57–74.

Part VI

Human guinea pigs and miracles: clinical innovations and unorthodox treatment

21

Amputate my arm, please. I don't want it anymore

Denise M. Dudzinski

Case narrative

I learned about Cindy during my routine attendance at multidisciplinary rounds. By attending rounds, I try to assist with emerging ethical issues before they become dilemmas and identify areas of ethical concern for resident physicians and other healthcare providers for discussion and education in various forums, both formal and informal. The resident physician gave me a basic history that prompted me to follow up on this patient.

Cindy Johnson is a 50-year-old woman who, 10 years ago, injured her wrist while working on an assembly line. Since the injury she has suffered from complex regional pain syndrome (CRPS) of her left hand and forearm. CRPS is a neuropathic pain disorder that arises after painful trauma affecting the limbs, a bone fracture, or as a consequence of stroke, spinal cord injury, or myocardial infarction.[1,2] Since even a gentle breeze passing over Cindy's exposed skin causes excruciating pain and a burning sensation, she keeps her forearm protected with a bandage and a hard brace. She often rests her arm on a pillow – a minor protection and a visible sign to others to keep their distance. Cindy was admitted through the emergency department after seeking a continuous infusion of levobupivacaine to anesthetize her arm shortly after a dressing change. This was her first dressing change in over a year. Due in part to suboptimal hygienic management, she suffers from cellulitis and edema in her left hand and forearm. She also has joint contractures in her left hand and her muscles have atrophied from lack of use. Without more frequent dressing changes her cellulitis will spread, causing ulcers and recurrent infections. Despite Cindy's past cooperation with psychiatric, palliative, and physical therapies, her pain continues. Cindy now refuses all proposed treatments and requests amputation.

A version of this chapter was originally published in *The Journal of Clinical Ethics*, 16(3): 196–201. ©2005 by *The Journal of Clinical Ethics*. Used with permission. All rights reserved.

Given this background, I decide to be involved. When I ask Cindy if she would mind speaking with me, she is receptive, willingly telling her story and answering my questions. Cindy describes a crisis of corporeal and personal integrity. She tells me, "This arm just gets in the way. I'm sick of being careful with it and telling everyone else to watch out. I can't play with my grandson for fear of bumping into him. If it's gone I won't worry about that anymore." When I ask her if her husband and children agree with amputation, she offers a knowing smile. She has been asked this question before.

She says, "They wish I didn't have to do it, but they see how much I've been suffering. No one can assure me the other treatments will cure my pain either, at least not without side effects I don't want to live with. It's a risk but it's what I want. And my family supports me."

Cindy lives with her husband and cares for her 5-year-old grandson, James. She is existentially and physically exhausted by constant pain and her inability to properly clean and protect her arm. Her inpatient team of physicians, including general medicine, psychiatry, pain service, and anesthesia, had presented several treatment options. These included intrathecal opioids, a spinal cord stimulator, and dorsal rhizotomy (cutting the spinal nerve roots). Cindy does not want the dorsal rhizotomy because her face will droop and she may experience numbness on her left side. She is not a candidate for spinal cord stimulator because she has too many nerves and the contractures in her hand are a contraindication.

Cindy refuses all proposed treatments and requests amputation. Her physicians warn that amputation will probably not alleviate the pain because phantom pain is likely to continue. Cindy wants amputation for hygienic and personal reasons. She will take the risk of phantom pain. Her arm is alien to her and is negatively impacting the quality of her relationships, especially her relationship with her grandson. The child is perpetually afraid he will hurt his grandma.

The treating physicians repeatedly spoke with Cindy about treatment alternatives and the risks of amputation. Cindy consistently assured them that she understood that amputation was unlikely to alleviate her pain. Whereas Cindy was certain, members of the team (including myself) were uncertain about whether amputation was medically or ethically appropriate or beneficial. As we grappled with the ethical dimensions of the case, we asked ourselves the following questions. Was her decisional capacity compromised by desperation? Was amputation a reasonable elective treatment alternative? Do harms outweigh benefits for Cindy? If so, should surgeons refuse her requests for amputation? Whose perspective should take precedence – the medical team's or Cindy's?

Haunting aspects

Ethics consultants, like their partners in consultation, experience moral distress and disequilibrium as well as remarkable opportunities for moral and professional growth. "Faced with intense, specific, and explicit attention to the actual circumstances, to the genuine agony and potential disruption encountered by vulnerable patients and their loved ones, and by clinicians, the ethics consultant's own sensibilities and judgments may undergo a kind of disequilibrium."[3] My involvement in Cindy's case produced a subtle disequilibrium that arises from critical reflection and the belated acknowledgment that I should have done better.

First, I am haunted because in retrospect I see that my moral distress took center stage. I was so relieved when Cindy assured me that amputation was best for her. Her assurance was a gift. Cindy's conviction made amputation, an irreversible intervention unlikely to alleviate her chief complaint, ethically permissible. With that assurance the case was closed for me and many members of the treating team. Was this the "respect for autonomy" trump card? Did I find it easier to agree with Cindy because doing so would relieve my moral distress? Cindy may truly be harmed by amputation. That reality did not change with my relief or her conviction. My distress arose not because I was haunted by the outcome but because I saw that the process was flawed.

Second, I am haunted by the fact that evidence suggests I did little to help. In fact, I might very well have contributed to Cindy's distress. Despite my attempts to be nonthreatening and to let her know that she did not have to speak with me, she probably perceived me as another institutional hurdle to clear before someone would grant her wish. She had to tell a painful story to yet another stranger. After living in pain for so long, why should she have to speak to an ethicist when her discussions with her doctors were genuinely ethically productive? Also, because there was no formal consult, I did not speak with all the people struggling with the decision to amputate. If I had truly wanted to help my colleagues, I would have spoken with more of them.

Third, I failed to recognize clear conflicts of interest. I had almost nothing to lose and a lot to gain from talking with Cindy. She might quell my curiosity and address my uncertainty. My conversation with Cindy benefited me professionally as well. I have added a valuable teaching case to my repertoire. At the end of our pleasant conversation in which we discussed both her values and the ethical concerns of the treating team, I asked Cindy if I could use her case for teaching. She agreed without hesitation. Even in retrospect I do not think I exploited Cindy, but I was not as sensitive as I should have been. Was I trying to make myself useful to the medical team, blind to the price (however small) to Cindy? Probably, since I was new to the institution and wanted to make a good impression. I wanted to be an interested, collaborative, and proactive ethicist with a gentle and respectful demeanor.

Professional reflections

A formal ethics consultation was never called. Hence, my role was not to help facilitate resolution of a conflict as it is in formal ethics consultation.[4] The process of moral deliberation had begun among those with most at stake. The deliberation was proceeding as one would expect – physicians were talking to one another and the patient, trying to decide what was best.[5] After talking with the resident physician after rounds, I asked the attending physician, Dr. Miriam Lam, if she would mind if I talked with Cindy about her choice. Dr. Lam welcomed my involvement as the treating team was divided about how to proceed. Still, my involvement was unsolicited. So why involve myself in this case?

First, I want ethics consultation to be more proactive than reactive. By making this shift, we can focus on giving providers the skills to address ethical issues and spend our time supporting staff, patients, and families in their ethical deliberations. This strategy is better than sweeping in at the final hour when an avoidable dilemma has arisen. Hence, informal consultations are routine in my practice, but informal consultations usually do not involve visiting patients since I am most often responding to healthcare provider concerns about ethical dimensions of patient care.

Second, I wanted to help. Vulnerable patients call out for a special kind of attention and care, inspiring a desire to protect. I feel this desire strongly. While I am intellectually aware of the dangers, the sentiment remains. The desire to protect, especially in the role of a clinical ethics consultant, can lead to meddling and ineffective consultation. Rather than focusing on facilitating conflict resolution, excavating shared values, and collaboratively envisioning creative solutions, one can become distracted by the drive of one's own conviction.

Any question of Cindy's decision-making capacity was motivated by her unusual request, not unclear thinking. She knew what she wanted to the point that she proposed an unorthodox treatment plan. She was vulnerable because she was trapped in her own body and only a surgeon could "save" her. While clinicians worried that amputation was elective disfigurement that would not alleviate her pain, Cindy thought of amputation as liberation. Her arm had become alien to her, marked by a sustained disruption to her sense of self because of a disruption in the relationships that shape her.[6,7,8] She experienced a crisis of corporeal integrity. She wanted to be free.

The third reason I became involved was because I was curious. Cindy's particular vulnerability has intrigued me for some time.[8] How do people learn to live with an illness or injury that forces them to change their very notion of themselves? Corporeal and personal integrity are radically challenged, and these patients courageously find and re-create themselves. I admire them and want to hear their stories. While I have no problem asking patients to teach us, in Cindy's case I was inexcusably unaware of how my own curiosity and professional self-interest compelled my involvement. At the end of our conversation, I asked Cindy if I could tell her story, especially in my work teaching residents. She willingly agreed and my interests once again prevailed. I believed at the time my involvement was more about wanting to help, but there was a clear conflict of interest.

Finally, I became involved because I wanted to help the treating team deal with its moral distress. By report, Cindy sounded desperate and absolutely convinced that amputation was best. Maybe by speaking with her I would better understand the paradox and quench my desire to help. We genuinely did not know what was best to do. We all wanted to be certain. Once again, I should not have been seduced by the comfort of certitude. The moral life entails living with uncertainty – doing what we think is best without the benefit of knowing if our actions will bring the good we desire. Ethicists collaborate with others to bring clarity to a complex situation, but striving for clarity does not mean striving for certainty. Maybe I had confused the two.

Moral distress is itself a kind of haunting. Moral distress arises when we identify the right course of action but feel constrained to act upon it.[9,10,11,12] Likewise, moral uncertainty breeds moral distress. Moral uncertainty is marked by nebulous, negative feelings or "warning" intuitions experienced when individuals have not yet identified the source of their discomfort. Moral uncertainty can be addressed by gathering more information and by clarifying and naming the source of distress. In Cindy's case, our moral distress arose from moral uncertainty.

Moral distress influences professional integrity because it is a visceral response to a conflict between our personal values and our professional obligations.[13,14] If our primary obligation is to help patients restore the personal integrity jeopardized by illness and injury, acceding to Cindy's request is ethically warranted. But if Cindy's request for amputation conflicts with the professional or personal values of healthcare providers, then a challenge to professional integrity arises.[6] If we do not believe that amputation is beneficial, should we condone it even if Cindy believes it is her best option? Doesn't this compromise our own integrity? If we do not actively discourage amputation, have we failed Cindy?

The attending physician, Dr. Miriam Lam, resolved her moral distress by talking with Cindy. She said, "As I talked to healthcare providers and Cindy, I felt ambivalent. I wasn't sure what was best to do and this troubled me. Amputating an arm is irreversible! What if she changes her mind? What if her pain gets worse? At first I wasn't sure what we should do. But that slowly changed. The more I talked with Cindy, the more I felt amputation was right for her. And I just accepted that it was my job as her doctor to do what was right for her even if I didn't completely understand." Cindy's clear expression of her wish to amputate assured Miriam.

Cindy's clear, consistent, autonomous request did not assure everyone. Several surgeons refused to amputate, citing a conflict with nonmaleficence and beneficence obligations. Some providers in pain and psychiatric services also disagreed with amputation. Amputation was not medically indicated for treating CRPS. Surgeons had no obligation to amputate, but ONLY a surgeon could grant Cindy her wish.

After speaking with Cindy I came to the same conclusion as Miriam. Cindy knew what she was doing and what was best for her. While individual surgeons may refuse to operate, I believed amputation was ethically permissible given that she understood the possible repercussions. Had I succumbed to the lure of a patient's informed, autonomous request – the autonomy trump card? There are at least two ways to think about the dilemma. On the one hand, we should trust the decisional patient's thoughtful assessment of harms and benefits when she suffers from a disability that negatively impacts the quality of her relationships. On the other hand, her physicians are obligated to minimize harm or to provide benefit, neither of which was expected from the perspective of care providers. At most an amputation would be a zero-sum gain, leaving her in the same pain but without an arm. To this day, I think favoring Cindy's assessment of benefit over a more objective "medical benefit" was ethically justifiable, but reasonable people will disagree on this point, particularly if they believe that Cindy's pain compromised her decision-making capacity. I do not believe this was the case, especially because a psychiatric assessment confirmed her decision-making capacity.

Outcome

One surgeon agreed to operate after several declined. Cindy did not experience any major complications from surgery, although several years after her surgery she continues to be treated for pain. How is Cindy doing now? Was amputation best for her? Does she regret it? How is her relationship with her grandson? I honestly do not know. I have not spoken with her since her hospitalization years ago.

Discussion questions

1. What would you do differently in this case? Why?
2. What are the consultant's obligations to Cindy? To her healthcare providers?
3. How is an informal consultation different from a formal consultation? Does the designation formal or informal impact standards of practice or our responsibilities to those involved in the case? Why or why not?
4. How can conflict of interest best be managed when writing about or teaching a "case"?
5. Should we seek consent when we teach or write about patients and providers? Why or why not?

REFERENCES

1. Wasner G, Backonja MM, Baron R. Traumatic neuralgias: Complex regional pain syndromes (reflex sympathetic dystrophy and causalgia): Clinical characteristics, pathophysiological mechanisms and therapy. *Neurol Clin*, 1998; 16: 851–68.
2. Wasner G, Schattschneider J, Binder A, Baron J. Complex regional pain syndrome – diagnostic, mechanisms, CNS involvement and therapy. *Spinal Cord*, 2003; 41: 61–75.

3. Bliton MJ, Finder SG. Traversing boundaries: Clinical ethics, moral experience, and the withdrawal of life supports. *Theor Med*, 2002; 23: 233–58.

4. Consultations TFoSfB. *Core Competencies for Health Care Ethics Consultation.* Glenview, IL: American Society for Bioethics and Humanities; 1998.

5. Dudzinski D. The practice of a clinical ethics consultant. *Public Aff Q*, 2003; 17(2): 121–39.

6. Pellegrino EDDCT. *The Virtues in Medical Practice.* Oxford: Oxford University Press, 1993.

7. Zaner RM. *The Context of Self: A Phenomenological Inquiry Using Medicine as a Clue.* Athens: Ohio University Press, 1981.

8. Dudzinski D. The diving bell meets the butterfly: Identity lost and remembered. *Theor Med Bioeth*, 2001; 22: 33–46.

9. Tiedje LB. Moral distress in perinatal nursing. *J Perinat Neonatal Nurs*, 2000; 14(2): 36–43.

10. Hefferman PSH. Giving "moral distress" a voice: Ethical concerns among neonatal intensive care unit personnel. *Camb Q Healthc Ethics*, 1999; 8: 173–8.

11. Sundin-Huard DKF. Moral distress, advocacy and burnout: Theorising the relationships. *Int J Nurs Pract*, 1999; 5: 8–13.

12. Erlen JA. Moral distress: A pervasive problem. *Orthop Nurs*, 2001; 20(2): 76–80.

13. Andre J. *Bioethics as Practice.* Chapel Hill: The University of North Carolina Press, 2002.

14. Benjamin M. Philosophical integrity and policy development in bioethics. *J Med Philos*, 1990; 15(4): 375–89.

22

Feuding surrogates, herbal therapies, and a dying patient

Alissa Hurwitz Swota

Case narrative

Ethics consultations typically share common characteristics. For instance, they are often called when conflict is already full-blown, when discord exists between surrogates and the healthcare team, and when there are disparities between the accounts of patient preferences given by surrogates. This case reflected all of these traits. However, deeply entrenched tensions combined with periods of profound sadness and misunderstanding made the case more complicated.

I participated in this consult while completing a postdoctoral fellowship in clinical ethics. I worked on the case with the full-time bioethicist for a large community hospital where I was doing a rotation. What follows is an abbreviated version of a complex case that took place over a couple of months.

Mr. Nelson was an 87-year-old man with metastatic cancer and dementia. Prior to being admitted to the palliative-care unit, Mr. Nelson had been admitted to a medicine floor after being found unconscious on the floor of his home. Mr. Nelson had given power of attorney for health care to his son and daughter to share equally, though his daughter was his primary caregiver.[1]

While on the medicine floor Mr. Nelson was found to be incapable of making treatment decisions, probably due to the metastases in his brain. After being transferred to the palliative-care unit, Mr. Nelson remained confused and cried a good portion of the time. Due to a fractured right hip that occurred when he fell at home, Mr. Nelson evidenced pain when he was moved.

The relationship between healthcare surrogates was strained at best, full of deep and long-standing conflict that carried over to the treatment plan and healthcare team. From the outset, Mr. Nelson's daughter accepted her father's extremely poor prognosis and was supportive of the medical team's plan to focus on palliative care. Conversely, his son was unwilling to believe that his father's condition would worsen progressively. He sought complete control over his father's treatment and maintained that his father would get "100% better" once the "poison" (pain and antipsychotic medications) was gone from his body.

Early on, Mr. Nelson's son requested that he be the one to feed his father breakfast. This seemed like a wonderful opportunity for father and son to interact. Unfortunately, in several instances Mr. Nelson's son was late, and his son demanded that the staff wait for him to feed his father. The healthcare team grew frustrated and angry as it watched Mr. Nelson wait longer and longer for his breakfast. Eating was one thing that still gave Mr. Nelson pleasure, and to make him wait for so long verged on cruelty.

Mr. Nelson's daughter was most disturbed that her brother, in the hope of prolonging and improving the quality of their father's life, gave their father herbal therapies while opposing the use of standard pain medication. Mr. Nelson's son believed his dad was a "fighter" who would not want to just "give up." The herbal therapies were his way of helping his dad battle cancer. When Mr. Nelson was first admitted to the palliative-care unit, his daughter agreed to allow her brother to administer the herbal therapies *alongside* standard pain medication. Fragile from the start, this accord unraveled as Mr. Nelson's son continued his push to stop standard pain medications. At the same time, concerns about the use of herbal therapies mounted. In light of these concerns, the healthcare team and Mr. Nelson's son held a meeting. A hospital pharmacist investigated all of the herbal therapies. The pharmacist made it clear to Mr. Nelson's son that there was insufficient evidence to support the effectiveness of herbal therapies, that they had an extensive list of possible side effects, and that it was unknown what effect they might have on his father at present doses and concentrations. Mr. Nelson's son remained steadfast in his resolve to continue giving his father the herbal therapies. Soon after this meeting, Mr. Nelson's son demanded that his father receive absolutely no standard pain medications. At this point, Mr. Nelson's daughter refused to sign the consent forms that allowed her brother to continue to administer the herbal therapies. She maintained that he had given them to their mother at the end of her life. Mr. Nelson had not been in favor of the herbal therapies for his wife and would not be in favor of receiving them if he were able to speak for himself.

Both Mr. Nelson's daughter and the healthcare team were uncomfortable with Mr. Nelson's son making unilateral decisions for his father. His sister did, after all, share equal power of attorney for health care for her father. Mr. Nelson's son resorted to threats of litigation at one point to gain complete control over the care of his father. Members of the healthcare team were doing their best to respect Mr. Nelson's son's difficult situation, accommodating his abrasive demeanor and constant demands in a calm, professional manner. At the same time, members of the healthcare team continued to care for Mr. Nelson and to help him avoid any unnecessary suffering at the end of his life. To be sure, this was no small feat. When nurses began to feel threatened and afraid to administer standard pain medications a bioethics consultation was requested.

After going to see Mr. Nelson, who seemed to be in distress and unable to participate in medical-treatment decisions, we met with his son and daughter –

separately of course. The siblings had very different goals and conflicting ideas of what their father's treatment plan should look like. We went over the philosophy of the palliative-care unit – to support and to care for patients while focusing on the quality of life for patients whose prognosis is less than three months – as a reminder of what everyone had signed on for when placing Mr. Nelson in this particular unit. This philosophy had been explained to Mr. Nelson and his family on numerous occasions. Each time *everyone* agreed to, understood, and was in favor of such care. Our explanation met with the same unanimous agreement. We also informed Mr. Nelson's son of the hospital's pain policy and told him that the nurses had a duty to help alleviate suffering. As such, they would continue to administer pain medications.

Each day I would go to the unit to see how things were progressing. Often members of the healthcare team would stop me. They shared stories of frustration after taking care of Mr. Nelson and expressed anxiety over having to care for him in the future. Frequently, members of the nursing staff would comment on how poorly Mr. Nelson's son treated his sister. They described Mr. Nelson's son as abrasive and overbearing, a bully both to them and to his sister. On the other hand, they saw Mr. Nelson's daughter as a victim, weak and in need of protection. Though ultimately I understood the basis for these descriptions, these preset characterizations compounded the already-difficult task of remaining objective when walking into a highly charged conflict. It was clear that the nursing staff had become distracted by what was happening between Mr. Nelson's son and daughter, and that, to a certain extent, they lost sight of the fact that the primary focus was Mr. Nelson's needs and interests.

As Mr. Nelson's son became more difficult and his contentious relationship with his sister continued to distract the medical-care team, we attempted to get the two decision-makers together to facilitate a smoother decision-making process and to refocus the care team. We recommended that they seek counseling. When recommending counseling, we made it clear to both surrogates that if things did not improve we were willing to go to court to revoke their power of attorney for health care. After they agreed to counseling, we set up appointments with a counselor in the hospital. For her first appointment, I escorted Mr. Nelson's daughter and sat with her in the waiting room. Our goal was to fix the siblings' relationship enough to enable them to work together to care for their father.

Against this backdrop, the other bioethicist and I worked to clarify roles, defuse power struggles, and help Mr. Nelson's children care for their father in their own way. All the while, we made sure to stay focused on Mr. Nelson's interests. Throughout my involvement in the case, I was struck by how certain each of the surrogates was about what their father would want and yet how drastically their accounts diverged. I was also concerned about the toll the case was taking on the members of the healthcare team who had to practice medicine and care for their patient under constant pressure and attempts by Mr. Nelson's son to usurp power.

It was clear to me that everyone involved was resigned to the idea that the best achievable outcome would be one of several poor options. I was disappointed in myself for setting what I thought was a very low goal. Even more, I was afraid that things were so bad even such a meager goal might not be met.

Professional reflections

First, it was clear that the differences between surrogates ran deep, with brother and sister diverging on basic ideas of what "caring" for their father meant and what a "good death" would look like for him. As a result, a large portion of the first meeting the other bioethicist and I had with the siblings was spent on conceptual clarification and determining what they understood the goals of treatment to be. When asked what was entailed in caring for her father, Mr. Nelson's daughter painted a picture in which her dad was comfortable and all efforts were directed toward that end. She described a "good death" as simply "peaceful." In contrast, Mr. Nelson's son explained that "caring" for his father meant exhausting any and all possibilities for keeping his dad alive and explained that *if* his dad were to die, a "good death" would be one in which his dad was "not out of it" and continued to fight until the end. He said that his dad had beat cancer before and could do it again. We attempted to negotiate with the siblings and figure out a treatment plan around which we could build consensus. Ultimately, Mr. Nelson's pain medicines were decreased a bit to see if this would still allow for proper pain management while at the same time allowing him to be a bit more lucid. All of this was done with the understanding that managing pain was the primary concern and that the pain medications would be increased at the discretion of the healthcare team. Several members of the healthcare team voiced concern that giving herbal therapies in place of standard pain medications would be a clear violation of the principle of nonmaleficence.

Every member of the healthcare team thought Mr. Nelson's son was perverting the role of a surrogate.[2] The role of a healthcare surrogate is to carry out the patient's wishes, or where these are not known, to act in the patient's best interest. In this case, the surrogates' accounts were contradictory, with support for both sides reduced to one surrogate's word against the other. In addition, the primary request from Mr. Nelson's son to discontinue proven standard pain medications and replace them with herbal therapies was contraindicated. Such requests led members of the healthcare team to question the motives of Mr. Nelson's son. Specifically, was he dictating a treatment plan for his father based on what *he* wanted for his father rather than on what was in his father's best interest or on what his father would have wanted if he had been able to speak for himself? Unfortunately, explaining the role of a healthcare surrogate made momentary differences at best with Mr. Nelson's son. Old behaviors resurfaced within a day or so. And though the healthcare team went to great lengths to accommodate his requests, Mr. Nelson's son was not satisfied with anything but complete compliance with *his* treatment plan.

The equal division of decision-making authority between the two children further complicated matters. Even in the best of circumstances such equal division of authority can lead to conflict. In this case we were working against a backdrop of long-standing conflicts between the two surrogates. I found myself getting angry at Mr. Nelson, who watched these conflicts between his children grow over the years and yet still chose to grant them equal authority. Lacking any documentation regarding Mr. Nelson's treatment preferences, the surrogates were left to develop a treatment plan based on whether the benefits of accepting/rejecting a treatment were outweighed by the burdens. Remaining constant through this process was the primacy placed on pain management. I am still not certain what Mr. Nelson would have wanted. Would he have wanted to remain on high doses of pain medications, forsaking lucidity for comfort? Would he have wanted to "fight 'till the end" with as much clarity as possible even in the face of great pain? Uncertainty on this matter left us to do the best we could to reconcile the contrasting accounts given by feuding surrogates.

Haunting aspects

I am taken by feelings of regret and uncertainty when I look back on this case. First, the professionals involved in the case were some of the best I have ever worked with. Given the unit they were on, they had a lot of experience caring for patients and their families at the end of life. I hoped that my presence and availability increased the likelihood that the moral distress of the healthcare team could be converted into a "teachable moment." My position as a fellow afforded me the luxury of dedicating extensive time to this particular case. At the same time, since I was a fellow and not the hospital bioethicist, there was uncertainty with regard to the boundaries within which I was operating, especially when it came to the extent (or lack thereof) of my authority to make recommendations. And though the whole team seemed grateful for my help, I still feel as though I did not do enough to lessen the stress experienced by the medical team.

Second, I am unsure whether we overstepped our boundaries as ethics consultants when we recommended and scheduled appointments for both surrogates to go to counseling. If we did, I am not sure it was a bad thing. Is scheduling counseling for surrogate decision-makers a part of what a clinical ethicist is responsible for? I am not sure. In this case, for these siblings and for this healthcare team, it seemed to work. Still, I am haunted by the thought that we could have been seen as meddlers and risked losing the trust of involved parties.

Third, I am angry at myself for colluding with a process that took too long, during which time I fear that Mr. Nelson may have been in pain. There were times when

Mr. Nelson would have a seemingly permanent wince etched in his face, as if he were staring into the noonday sun. At these times I wanted to shake Mr. Nelson's son and show him that his father was in pain. The standard pain medications should have been increased and not discontinued in favor of unproven herbal therapies. I wanted to plead with him to work harder to find common ground with his sister, if for nothing else than to show his father that they could work together. At the same time I am angry at myself for becoming so enraged and not remaining objective. I wish I could have done more, though I am not sure what, to speed up the facilitation process.

Outcome

Mr. Nelson died on the day of his children's first counseling sessions. His daughter was at his bedside and his son had just left the hospital. When his son received word that his father had died he was devastated, not only because of the news itself but also because he was not at his father's side. At once his hard, abrasive, arrogant demeanor changed and he was simply someone who had just lost his dad. News of Mr. Nelson's death came as something of a relief to me. I was relieved not only because Mr. Nelson was no longer in pain but also because the demoralized healthcare team would gain reprieve from such a difficult case. A couple of days after Mr. Nelson died I received a thank you card from the healthcare team. I still have that card years later. I am not sure if I keep it because it somehow validated my work on the case or because it reminds me of how hard I must work in the future so I might have fewer regrets.

Discussion questions

1. Did the bioethicists overstep their boundaries in setting up counseling for the surrogates? If yes, was it a bad thing?
2. What more could have been done to speed up the decision-making process?
3. What place, if any, do herbal therapies have in the care of patients? Is their use more/less acceptable at the end of life?
4. Are labels placed on patients and families by healthcare providers ever useful? Can they act as shorthand for information or do they always negatively predispose the consultant?

ACKNOWLEDGMENTS

The author wishes to acknowledge Doreen Ouellet and Bonnie Steinbock for their gracious editorial assistance.

REFERENCES

1. For further details concerning power of attorney for health care as alluded to in this case, see Canada's Health Care Consent Act. Available at http://www.e-laws.gov.on.ca/DBLaws/Statutes/English/96h02_e.htm
2. Legislation on advance directives will vary between states, but a nice explanation of advance directives and how they function is available at http://www.icare.ws/modules/Module10.pdf. In particular, see A.17: Can a Power of Attorney Be Revoked or Modified?

23

One way out: destination therapy by default

Alice Chang and Denise M. Dudzinski

Case narrative

A year before Rose was admitted, Alice (the heart transplant social worker and a clinical ethics consultant) and her team invited Denise (chief of the ethics consultation service and an organizational ethics consultant) to explore the ethical dimensions of a new treatment called destination therapy (DT). The Randomized Evaluation of Mechanical Assistance for Treatment of Congestive Heart Failure (REMATCH) study showed that an LVAD (left ventricular assist device, which is surgically implanted to do the work of a poorly functioning left ventrical) can prolong life and decrease morbidity for patients with advanced cardiac disease who are not candidates for transplant.[1,2] For this group, the LVAD is "destination" rather than "bridge" therapy. The target population was the estimated 10% of heart failure patients older than 65 with refractory end-stage heart failure, not young patients like Rose.[3] By the time Rose was admitted, the heart transplant team, Alice, and Denise had worked together for months and had drafted ethics guidelines.[4] Unfortunately, these did not help Rose at all.

Rose was a woman in her late 20s with severe cardiomyopathy and very poor cardiac function (ejection fraction <10%). She was admitted to the hospital to receive treatment for congestive heart failure symptoms, including shortness of breath, nausea, vomiting, and general malaise. Because she was so acutely ill, she received an expedited transplant workup that revealed no major medical contraindications but highlighted several psychosocial "red flags" that included a history of substance abuse, previous nonadherence to medical regimen, and lack of insurance and stable social support. Rose frequently missed clinic appointments and did not always take her medicines as prescribed. For a variety of reasons, including her young age, she may not have fully understood the severity of her disease. The transplant team planned to help Rose address some of these issues, but then she faced a medical crisis.

To save her life one Saturday morning, an LVAD was placed emergently before the transplant team had made a final listing decision. LVAD patients are tethered to a small refrigerator-sized contraption in the hospital (as in Rose's case initially) or to a more portable LVAD if a long wait for transplant is anticipated and the patient can live outside the hospital. Usually a listing decision *precedes* LVAD placement. Her emergent LVAD implantation meant she would have to be considered for a transplant because she was too young to meet the REMATCH criteria for DT. If she did not eventually meet transplant criteria, she would become a DT patient by default.

Given Rose's tragic story, the medical team felt a heightened need to take care of her. Rose spent her childhood in foster homes because her mother struggled with heroin addiction. She was sexually abused in her early teens. One rape resulted in a pregnancy. Rose gave birth at the age of 15, and her newborn daughter was adopted by parents who allowed Rose to correspond with her child. This was the bright spot in Rose's life. Rose said, "I don't have a good relationship with my mom, no education, no money. It makes my day when I see cards and prayers from my daughter and her family. That's all I have. It's what I live for some days."

When Rose turned 18, she was homeless and periodically supported herself through prostitution, blunting her grief with drugs and alcohol. When Rose was 20 she reconnected with her mother. There was hope that her social network would improve. During Rose's initial hospitalization in the intensive-care unit, her mother visited every day and promised to be her primary caregiver after the transplant. (A committed primary caregiver is required to move forward with transplant.)

Rose recovered well physically from the LVAD surgery in the following weeks, but she was anxious and irritable. The psychiatry service started seeing her daily and diagnosed major depression and anxiety disorder, both linked to her feelings of isolation, her poor coping mechanisms, and her difficulty bonding with others. Psychiatry followed her until she was finally released 6 months later with a portable LVAD. LVAD patients need close observation by family to manage emergencies. Her mother and a number of friends were trained in how the LVAD worked and were advised about how to help Rose if it malfunctioned. They would take turns caring for her. Unfortunately, Rose's relationship with her mother was volatile. Verbal altercations escalated to physical threats.

Three weeks later, after missing her outpatient mental health appointments, Rose was readmitted to the hospital for lack of support in the community. Her mother's care was inconsistent at night and various friends were unreliable during the day. The only safe place for Rose seemed to be the hospital. Soon after admission, Rose's mother stepped down as Rose's caregiver, citing intractable conflict.

In addition to the justice issue raised by making the hospital her home absent medical necessity, the transplant team faced an additional ethical dilemma. Should they remove Rose from the transplant list, making Rose a "destination therapy" patient by default? Alice enlisted the help of the ethics consultant on-call (not Denise). Both consultants agreed that delisting was permissible because (a) it was consistent with the hospital's policy and with previous stipulations for listing Rose (it was fair, albeit heartbreaking), and (b) the harms of transplant without social support likely outweigh the benefits.

Rose was told she would be removed from the transplant list with the possibility of relisting if her adherence to medical and mental health treatment improved and if she could find a stable living situation with a consistent caregiver. Rose refused nursing home placement, and her last option was to move in with her new boyfriend, David. Rose planned to pool their resources and rent an apartment together. After one week of living together, David moved out, and Rose once again lost her caregiver, social support, and housing.

Rose became more depressed and requested weaning from the LVAD because she realized she would never find the social support she needed to qualify for a transplant. After a weaning attempt, Rose was told she could not be weaned off the machine because her heart could not function without it and she needed the device to keep her alive. Sometimes Rose would sit in the hospital lobby hoping to be admitted.

A week later, Rose overdosed on pain medication while living with Miriam, a respite caregiver with whom Rose was temporarily staying. She was seen in another hospital's emergency department, treated, and sent home. A week later, she turned off her LVAD when Miriam was in another room. Miriam reacted quickly and turned the LVAD back on. Rose was intubated and admitted to the intensive-care unit.

Professional reflections

At our institution, one clinical ethics consultant is on-call at all times and that person usually handles formal ethics consultations alone. In addition, many help with informal "preventive" ethics consultations by providing education and support for day-to-day ethical issues that arise in patient care. At weekly "selection conferences," the transplant team checks in with Alice to "make sure we're on firm [ethical] ground." As the social worker, Alice provided social support for Rose, identified ways to help her meet listing criteria, and outlined the nonmedical risks and benefits of transplantation. Alice wore two hats. There were three clinical ethics decision points when the team sought help from Alice.

First consultation: Should Rose be considered for transplant at all? From a psychosocial standpoint, high-risk transplant candidates include patients with prior history of nonadherence, past psychiatric admissions, presence of a mood or personality disorder, history of ongoing substance abuse and nicotine dependence, and lack of confirmed social support. These patients have much higher mortality rates, more than two-and-a-half-times greater than those classified as "acceptable" or "good" candidates.[5] Alice assessed Rose's risk as between acceptable and high at best.

Two controversial psychosocial risk factors for Rose were recent rehabilitated substance abuse and a history of nonadherence. There is considerable controversy about excluding patients for either of these reasons.[5,6] On the one hand, Rose's youth suggests she will be more resilient after transplant. However, without adherence to immunosuppressive drug regimens, diet, lifestyle restrictions (including eliminating nicotine, alcohol, and illicit drugs), close monitoring for signs of complications, and regular clinic follow-ups, Rose's graft will not thrive and neither will Rose.[7] The team planned to help Rose address these issues so she could be listed.

Alice said to the team, "If we do this today for Rose, we have to be willing to do the same with patients in similar circumstances tomorrow. Are we willing to do that?" The team was ambivalent and confounded. Alice sympathized but suspected life posttransplant would be very difficult for Rose. Medical treatment cannot fix entrenched social problems. Alice did not recommend listing her initially, but then Rose "crashed" on a weekend.

Second consultation: After Rose received her LVAD, Alice worried that in the interest of saving Rose the team had actually sealed her tragic fate. This raised an ethical question. By placing an LVAD emergently (and therefore provisionally listing her for transplant) was the team consistently following its own listing guidelines? The surgeon said, "She was so young. I just wasn't ready to throw in the towel when she was crashing." The hope was that she would "perk up" medically, be discharged, and have time to meet listing criteria by (a) undergoing substance abuse assessment and treatment (this proved unnecessary), (b) demonstrating adherence to medical treatment, (c) not missing clinic appointments, and (d) identifying reliable social supports. This seemed to be the fairest approach, but it was fraught with "ifs." Ironically, the team's commitment to helping Rose also probably set her up for failure. Alice and members of the transplant team continue to be haunted by this.

The DT ethics guidelines discourage emergent LVAD placement because it curtails informed consent.[4] To the patient it can look like a bait and switch: "They put the LVAD in so they must be planning to transplant me." The patient consents to transplant as cure, but when the team decides she is not a transplant candidate, the LVAD ticks on. She is a DT patient by "default" without her explicit consent. Alice was particularly concerned about "DT by default" patients. In emergencies, quick clinical judgments must be made, and NOT placing the LVAD would have seemed like discrimination and abandonment to the surgeon. Hence, more than a policy is necessary – a slow culture shift is needed. Rose's case set the culture shift in motion.

Third consultation: Alice and another ethics consultant (not Denise) conferred when the transplant team faced delisting Rose. Was it fair? Team members felt they were taking away her only "chance" and they were not fulfilling their "promise." However, any benefit Rose might enjoy would be linked to her social circumstances and overall quality of life, which was poor despite multiple attempts to help her improve it. Ultimately both consultants agreed delisting was ethically permissible because social support is required for all transplant patients and is essential to their health and well-being.

Haunting aspects

Alice and Denise both regret that, even at this point, palliative care was not more seriously considered. It was the obvious alternative, but the team continued to hold out hope that she could cobble together social support and be listed. Perhaps the prospect of turning off an LVAD was just too hard, too uncharted, too counter to the transplant culture. Talking in advance with patients about turning off the LVAD and then actually doing it would be stressful and emotionally trying for the team. It was outside of the transplant team's scope of normal practice and would engender moral confusion and distress.

The obligation to offer and provide palliative care was one of the major entreaties in the DT ethics guidelines we drafted. If we implant an LVAD, we should be prepared to turn it off and to help manage the patient's pain and symptoms. The team understood that patients have a right to withdraw treatments, but turning off an LVAD – a device anastomosed to the patient's heart – meant turning off the patient's heart. For some that seemed like euthanasia. Would Rose have taken all those pain pills or disconnected her LVAD if she had known that her doctors would support her decision to stop the LVAD? Was her suicide attempt a reflection of her depression or of her desire to stop burdensome treatment or both? Was this another example of Rose being abandoned? We are haunted by these unanswered questions.

For Alice, being the social worker and ethics consultant created moral distress. In wearing both hats, Alice felt "all alone," trying to "keep [her] head above the water." Every week the team talked about Rose and anguished over her candidacy for heart transplant. The team was hopeful she would meet transplant criteria and cognizant that the deck was stacked against her. The same questions swirled under the surface week after week. What are her options if we do not transplant her? What is her life going to be like? And we "did this to her." Should we follow through as a matter of loyalty or compassion? Was it fair to use LVAD as a bridge to transplant and then default to DT when "things" did not work out? The best hope was weaning. When that failed, the team felt like it had made her life hell no matter how it played out. Doubt and ambiguity prevailed, and Alice experienced that as a member of the treating team.

However, from a clinical ethics perspective, Rose did not meet criteria. The criteria are there in the interest of fairness and in recognition that transplantation is not an innocuous treatment. A lifetime of immunosuppression therapy and constant medical monitoring are facts of life for transplant patients, and the transplant professionals are stewards of scarce cadaveric organs. Justice requires treating like patients alike, but justice might also require "going the extra mile" for someone who has suffered so much for so long.

Alice also worried about the informed-consent process. Did we (the transplant team) provide enough information to Rose and her family about the benefits and burdens of LVAD therapy? Rose's status on the transplant list was never clear. It was always hoped that there was a remote chance she could be relisted. We were never on firm ground. Even the team never really knew whether Rose was truly a candidate for DT. If it was not clear to us, how could it be clear to Rose? Did we do justice by offering these choices knowing she had very limited resources? Or did we do the right thing by giving her a "fighting chance" despite the limitation? Rose answered this question by overdosing and disconnecting the LVAD. Rose should not have been all alone.

Because of her dual role, Alice was in a perpetual ethics consultation. I (Denise) was oblivious to the stress this caused Alice. I am haunted because I abandoned my colleague. Rose embodied the organizational ethics conundrum of DT. Caring for Rose provided the first occasion to test the ethics guidelines, but her story unfolded as if her situation was novel and unexpected. I failed to see the emotional and moral experiences of team members as an ongoing organizational issue that needed proactive rather than reactive attention. Instead, everyone felt the tragedy and Rose had to live it. Each ethics consultation was too episodic and narrow in scope, as if the three ethics consultations were not linked. Out of habit, I looked for critical decision points for formal, clearly delineated ethics consultations. I did not want to "meddle," which allowed me to protect myself from the pain of being closely involved while leaving Alice to bear the burden without the support I owe her as chief of the ethics consultation service.

In the end, the most haunting aspect of this case is the sense that we abandoned Rose – every one of us. She died alone in an act of desperation. At the least, we should have prevented that.

Outcome

After turning off her LVAD, Rose was in a coma. The CT scan showed multiple brain infarcts suggesting dismal prospects for survival. Another clinical ethics consultation was requested before the LVAD was deactivated once and for all. The treating physician wanted to be sure no one opposed deactivation. This was a new predicament for everyone. The LVAD was discontinued and Rose died in the intensive-care unit with her family at her side. Because of Rose, the transplant team is more circumspect about DT and speaks more openly about palliative-care options earlier in the process. The guidelines remain unchanged and practitioners are slowly becoming more accepting of the prospect of "withdrawing" an LVAD.

After Rose's death, a clinician who cared for Rose stopped Denise in the hall and said with sadness and regret, "What you said might happen did happen" (i.e., the patient turned the device off without medical assistance, pain, or symptom management). It will haunt all of us forever.

Discussion questions

1. What steps could have been taken to make sure the DT guidelines were actually going to be helpful?
2. What kind of organizational and clinical ethics support do you think clinicians need when they embark on innovative therapies?
3. How morally relevant are "emergencies" in deciding the implementation of innovative therapies when the emergency may be created, in part, by the patient's level of adherence?
4. What are strategies for convincing medical teams to prospectively create policies for rare but expected occurrences (i.e., not to wait for there to be a "Rose" case before addressing the ethical issues)?

REFERENCES

1. Rose EA, Gelijins AC, Moskowitz AJ, et al. (REMATCH Study Group). Long-term mechanical left ventricular assistance for end-stage heart failure. N Engl J Med, 2001; 345: 1435–43.
2. Rose EA, Moskowitz AJ, Packer M, et al. The REMATCH trial: Rationale, design, and end points. Ann Thorac Surg, 1999; 67(3): 723–30.
3. Lietz K, Miller LW. Will left-ventricular assist device therapy replace heart transplantation in the foreseeable future? Curr Opin Cardiol, 2005; 20: 132–7.
4. Dudzinski D. Ethics guidelines for destination therapy. Ann Thorac Surg, 2006; 81: 1185–8.
5. Owen JE, Bonds CL, Wellisch DK. Psychiatric evaluations of heart transplant candidates: Predicting post-transplant hospitalization, rejection episodes, and survival. Psychosomatics, 2006; 47(3): 213–22.
6. Levenson JL, Olbrisch ME. Psychosocial evaluation of organ transplant candidates. A comparative survey of process, criteria, and outcomes in heart, liver, and kidney transplantation. Psychosomatics, 1993; 34(4): 314–23.
7. De Geest S, Dobbels F, Fluri C, et al. Adherence to the therapeutic regimen in heart, lung, and heart–lung transplant recipients. J Cardiovasc Nurs, 2005; 20(5S): S88–S98.

24

Altruistic organ donation: Credible? Acceptable?

Ronald B. Miller

Case narrative

Mrs. Alberta "Allie" Truistic, a married mother of a 10-year-old and a 12-year-old, offered to donate a kidney to any patient with end-stage kidney disease who could benefit from transplantation. Having been refused by three transplant programs, she presented to a fourth in 1996. A thoughtful transplant surgeon in our university program asked me, a nephrologist and clinical ethicist, what he should do. I recommended he undertake a study of altruistic, nondirected, unrelated renal-transplant donation and consult the institutional review board (i.e., the human subjects research committee). He preferred to consult with the medical ethics committee of which I was vice chairman. The committee of 15 physicians, 8 nurses, 5 hospital administrators, 4 community representatives, 3 social workers, 3 bioethicists, and 2 attorneys performed ethics consultation either with a small team of four individuals or with the committee as a whole, as in this case.

The transplant surgeon told the committee that Allie Truistic had been motivated to donate ever since the death of her grandmother from polycystic kidney disease. She was told her grandmother, who had been on dialysis for several years, would have lived had she received a kidney transplant. Mrs. Truistic attended a meeting of our ethics committee and informed us that her husband and children supported her wish to donate. Concerned that detailed questioning by the 28 members of our committee might be intimidating, the transplant surgeon and two committee members (including the author) interviewed the patient. She was committed to donate and had a thorough understanding of the risks. She considered the possibility that one of her children could develop kidney disease and need a transplant and also that she could die from a complication, but she felt the gift of donation of a transplant was sufficient reward for her to take such risks. Upon rejoining the meeting in progress she told the interviewers and the two dozen ethics committee members that if only someone had donated a kidney to her grandmother she would not have died. Mrs. Truistic put us at ease concerning the potential for her children to inherit polycystic kidney disease by informing us that her "grandmother" was her husband's stepgrandmother (i.e., not a blood relative). This, together with a preliminary medical evaluation, demonstrated that the patient was likely a medically qualified donor, but what about psychologically and socially? Although the three of us who had interviewed her in detail were satisfied that she was emotionally healthy and appropriately motivated, the committee as a whole was highly suspicious. After the patient was thanked and excused from the meeting, the committee members posited that Allie Truistic either had a serious emotional disturbance or was seeking secondary gain and should have a psychiatric evaluation. A community member of the committee felt it was inappropriate to require all potential altruistic donors to have psychiatric evaluations. A thoughtful pediatrician recommended that Mrs. Truistic defer renal donation until her now 11- and 13-year-old children were two or three years older so they would be less severely affected if she were to die as a consequence of donation. A motion to approve the donation (if cleared after angiography and psychiatric evaluation) was tabled. The committee insisted it review the matter again after further testing and consultation.

The transplant surgeon consulted the United Network for Organ Sharing (UNOS), since altruistic donation was uncommon in 1997 despite the improvement in immunosuppressive pharmacology that had improved graft survival. To further test Mrs. Truistic's altruism, the transplant surgeon informed her there would be no press release or other publicity.

In early 1998, despite psychiatric clearance for donation, the ethics committee had not yet made a recommendation. Therefore, I moved that "the committee endorse and approve the anonymous, voluntary, informed donation" by Mrs. Truistic. The motion passed without dissent, but an administrator member of the ethics committee commented that we should have consulted a psychiatrist from an institution other than our own. The law professor-community member reiterated that in the future we should not require psychiatric examination unless there is a reason to question the competence of a potential altruistic donor. The author and another physician recommended that all potential living organ donors (segmental liver, lung, pancreas, or intestine as well as kidney) have a physician advocate who is not the physician of any potential recipient and who is not a member of the institution's transplant program.

UNOS recommended the donor organ be offered to recipients on the local waiting list unless there was an immunologically ideal (six-antigen) match elsewhere. The surgeon felt that for our first anonymous altruistic donor transplant the recipient should "be in sufficient health to benefit maximally from the transplant." The recipient pool was narrowed to those known to the institution. Finally, more than two years after Mrs. Truistic first offered donation to our institution and shortly after she proclaimed a deadline for a decision, her kidney was transplanted to "the first eligible recipient" on the institution's waiting list.

After the initial few months of follow-up, the transplant surgeon recommended Mrs. Truistic have lifelong, annual follow-up. When last seen four years after donation, Mrs. Truistic had stable renal function and remained proud of her donation. Subsequently she was lost to follow-up despite multiple attempts to locate her. Although she requested anonymity, she had given permission for scientific or professional discussion of her donation.

Haunting aspects

I am haunted by the professional distrust of altruism – or more properly the distrust of a person so willing to donate an organ anonymously. Perhaps I am more upset because I knew the distrustful members of our ethics committee were competent, selfless, healthcare professionals of integrity and compassion. But I believe their distrust was more than a simple paternalistic expression of fiduciary responsibility owed to patients, or in this case to a healthy woman willing to risk anesthesia, surgery, and life with a single kidney. Why did this woman wish to be a good samaritan? Should we really allow her to risk her own health simply for the benefit of another? Can we find a medical excuse to disqualify her? And, if not, will a psychiatrist take the rap for us by denying her request? There must be something wrong with her! But even if not, is informed consent really possible for someone who has not gone to medical or nursing school?

Why am I haunted? Many of us receive unconditional love from our parents and devoted care from nursery school and grade school teachers. We may be mentored by a friend of our parents, an athletic coach, or a librarian, yet we are suspicious of altruism even when we gratefully receive it ourselves. Too often we suspect psychiatric illness. The "altruistic" donor must be "crazy," must be seeking secondary gain, or must be engaged in occult black market dealings with the recipient. The distrust is not limited to ethics committees. It extends to psychiatrists, transplant surgeons, and some members of the public.[1,2]

I am haunted by healthcare professionals who think they know better than the patient what is right for the patient. We attempt to protect patients from themselves and to find medical rather than ethical excuses for disallowing altruistic organ donation. Perhaps we appear arrogant to our colleagues when we suggest that as members of ethics committees we are more appropriate decision-makers or gatekeepers than the attending physician who is traditionally the patient's advocate.

Professional reflections

This case has lessons for the conduct of ethics consultation as well as lessons regarding altruistic organ donation. I include comments regarding the latter because other ethics committees have struggled, or will struggle, with the issues of altruistic organ donation as well as with issues of organ donation after cardiac death.

Perhaps the most important lesson of this case is that we need to trust patients. This is the very meaning of "respect for persons." We need to understand that although altruistic donation is uncommon and "supererogatory," we should not presume that there is a psychopathological or abnormal motivation when an individual wishes to be a good samaritan. Caution is still warranted in response to offers of altruistic donation. A physician whose patients would not benefit personally from the altruistic donation should evaluate and advocate for the potential donor. Institutional policy should allow for due process and for appeal as appropriate. Ethics committees tend to be arbitrators, making decisions after hearing both sides of an issue. This may be reasonable in many circumstances, but when there is unresolved conflict, there may need to be consultation with extramural ethics committees, an extramural consultant, and/or a mediator.[3,4,5]

Another question is how to include patients and their families in ethics consultation and committee deliberation. This is relatively easy when there is a single consultant or a small consulting team, but it is much more threatening to a patient and family if they are interviewed by a large committee.[6] Furthermore, they may be inhibited by the presence of members of the patient-care team and vice versa such that one might consider limiting the number of people in the interview. However, in many circumstances it is important for the teams to hear each other, so there may be reasons to have both parties present throughout. Clearly there should not be an arbitrary and inflexible policy. Rather there should be adaptation to the specific circumstances planned by the individual who triages the ethics committee consultations. There are many more aspects that could be discussed (such as how to avoid conflicts of interest in ethics consultation and what counts as due process in ethics consultation), but I will focus on issues for altruistic organ donation.

Why was I the only member of our ethics committee willing to approve Alberta Truistic's initial offer to donate a kidney? Why did I believe her altruism was genuine and reasonable when others felt impelled to protect her from herself? I turned to the literature. To my surprise, neither altruistic kidney donation nor suspicion on the part of professionals was new.[1,2]

Despite my training in the early 1960s and subsequent practice and teaching of nephrology, I had forgotten the substantial numbers of kidneys altruistically donated in the late 1960s and early 1970s. I also had not read the literature so relevant to the issues troubling me three decades later. I was mistaken in believing – as many contemporary nephrologists also believe – that donation of kidneys from living but biologically unrelated individuals began with the recent development of more effective immune-suppressant medications.[7,8] Perhaps the first psychological study of living but unrelated kidney donors was that of Fellner and Marshall in the *Journal of the American Medical Association (JAMA)* in 1968[9] and in the *American Journal of Psychiatry* in 1970.[10] In 1971, Sadler, Davison, Carroll, and Kountz reported on living, genetically unrelated kidney donors, a study that began in 1967.[1] They focused on the ethical issues of such donation and created what was probably the first patient-care/research-subjects "ethics" committee years before the Quinlan case[11] popularized ethics committees for hospitals and prior to the introduction of institutional review boards for human subjects research.[12] They called their committee an "advisory panel." It consisted of a professor of theology, hermeneutics, and philosophy; a professor of law; and a professor of medical philosophy, Otto Guttengag. The authors studied 18 actual donors and 22 individuals who offered to donate but did not. They also surveyed 54 transplant centers and polled public opinion. They concluded that "use of the living, genetically unrelated donor as an organ source . . . is in all likelihood as moral as [use] of the cadaver donor . . . [and] is probably more moral than the use of the genetically related donor because of the reduced chances for his moral coercion as a result of his family position."[1] They stated "a voluntary, altruistic, and personally rewarding act of donating a kidney to an unrelated person is viewed by most physicians as impulsive, suspect, and repugnant – although the public does not share their view."[1]

One of the authors stated, "Perhaps the most dismaying feature of the response to the poll of transplant centers is the inherent suspicion of one's fellow men." (See page 99 of ref. 1.) Reports of the Human Renal Transplant Registry showed that "by the end of 1969 there had been . . . about 60 unrelated living donors who were not also spouses of the recipients or "free kidney" donors undergoing a mandatory nephrectomy" for a medical condition.[13] In 1971, Fellner and Schwartz titled an article in the *New England Journal of Medicine* about medical versus public attitudes toward the living organ donor "Altruism in Disrepute."[2] They noted that the famous French nephrologist Jean Hamburger implied that physician participation in altruistic donation "may be akin to a criminal rather than an ethical act."[2] In 1971, the International Transplantation Society issued a declaration that included the following statements: "The risk to the donor . . . must be a primary consideration, and the benefit to the recipient secondary. . . . We do not consider it necessary that a committee constituted of physicians and laymen should make such a judgment [the decision to accept a donor].[13] It is recognized that altruism on the part of the donor may be a real motivating factor and that the wish to donate an organ need not be a sign of mental instability."[13]

Despite this balanced statement and arguments on ethical grounds (potential harm to and impulsive rather than reflective decision making by living donors),[9,10,12] one might speculate that the change in attitudes (favoring cadaveric rather than living donor kidney transplantation) is related to the improved results of cadaveric donor transplantation and the widespread acceptance, following the Harvard ad hoc committee's report,[14] of death by neurologic criteria, which allowed a substantial decrease in cold ischemia time of the transplanted organ compared with the prior era when death was declared only on cardiopulmonary grounds. However, two reports in 1973[13,15] stated that genetically unrelated living volunteer donors were no longer being used in transplantation, and registry reports indicated the practice ended in 1969 (before most states had legalized death by neurologic criteria).[16] Fortunately for patients with end-stage kidney failure, deceased donor transplantation improved and dialysis became more available in the late 1960s, especially after Medicare entitlement (to dialysis and renal transplantation) became effective in 1973, reducing the need for living donors.[17]

Nevertheless, in 1986, Levey, Hou, and Bush called for reconsideration of the prohibition of unrelated living donation.[7] They did so because there were insufficient cadaveric donors, there were reasons to believe that the success of transplantation from living, unrelated donors "should be equal or superior to the success of cadaveric transplantation," and because the nephrectomy risks were thought to be minimal and the benefits sufficient to be ethically justified.[7] Attitudes changed, and Aaron Spital reported that 93% of transplant centers that responded to a 1999 survey "would accept a close friend as a kidney donor [and] although the majority of centers would not consider an altruistic stranger as a donor, a sizable minority (38%) would."[18] Furthermore, with immunosuppression improvements, living unrelated donor transplantation is as successful as living related donor transplantation.[19,20] There has been a progressive increase in the number of nondirected, living, unrelated donor transplants (from 1 in 1998 to 73 in 2003)[21] as well as an increase in directed but genetically unrelated living donor transplants (such as to a spouse). With increased success and increased number of nondirected, living, unrelated donor transplants, issues of ethical concern have changed. Most agree that donations to biologically unrelated recipients should be directed to spouses, other relatives, or friends but that donations may not be directed based on racial, gender, lifestyle, or other discriminatory criteria.[22,23,24,25,26] Ethical uncertainty remains. What if the organ is directed to a child or to a minority or another vulnerable group?[22,26] May organs be directed to one's own institution rather than to the regional or national waiting list? Do gifts of organs create moral obligations for recipients? What if the recipient does not reliably adhere to the immunosuppressive regimen? What are the long-term adverse health effects of organ donation? Contemporary ethics committees doing consultations for organ donation need to consider these issues.

Outcome

The transplant recipient has remained off dialysis and was most appreciative. The donor developed a hernia in the nephrectomy incision that required surgical repair, but she remained pleased for having donated. The transplant team was proud that anonymity was preserved and that it had performed one of the first anonymous, nondirected, altruistic living donor transplants in the modern era.

The ethics committee felt satisfied that it had deliberated carefully and that the delay had assured proper motivation of the donor. The consultation resulted in a hospital policy for anonymous living-kidney donation, as well as greater acceptance and less suspicion of altruistic donation and expeditious response to a subsequent altruistic donor. The author recognizes that a large, multidisciplinary ethics committee can explore ideas and options that might not be considered by a solo consultant or small team. However, there is also the risk of "group think" and delay, which in this case was unfair to the donor.

Discussion questions

1. Should patients or families attend ethics committee discussions of their case? If so, how much involvement should they have?
2. Is related (genetically, socially) living donor organ transplantation ethically permissible? Is altruistic, unrelated living donor kidney transplantation ethically permissible? Is one more ethical than the other?
3. If unrelated living donor kidney transplantation is ethically permissible, should the recipient be allowed to know the identity of, correspond with, or meet the donor?

REFERENCES

1. Sadler HH, Davison L, Carroll C, Kountz SL. The living genetically unrelated kidney donor. *Semin Psychiatry*, 1971; 3(1): 86–101.
2. Fellner CH, Schwartz SH. Altruism in disrepute: Medical versus public attitudes towards the living organ donor. *N Engl J Med*, 1971; 284(11): 582–5.
3. Miller RB. A call for regional ethics committees for ESRD patient problems. *Adv Ren Replace Ther*, 2000; 7(4): E5.
4. Miller RB. Extramural ethics consultation: Reflections on the mediation/medical advisory panel model and a further proposal. *J Clin Ethics*, 2002; 13(3): 203–15.
5. Miller RB. Mediation for challenging patients: A promising approach. *Adv Ren Replace Ther*, 1997; 4: 372–6.
6. Swenson MD, Miller RB. Ethics case review in health care institutions: Committees, consultants, or teams? *Arch Intern Med*, 1992; 152: 694–97.
7. Levey AS, Hou S, Bush HL Jr. Kidney transplantation from unrelated living donors: Time to reclaim a discarded opportunity. *N Engl J Med*, 1986; 314(14): 914–6.
8. Colaneri J. Living anonymous kidney donation: A solution to the organ donors shortage. "No, the research is incomplete." *Nephrol Nurs J*, 2004; 31(3): 330–1.
9. Fellner CH, Marshall JR. Twelve kidney donors. *JAMA*, 1968; 206(12): 2703–7.
10. Fellner CH, Marshall JR. Kidney donors – the myth of informed consent. *Am J Psychiatry*, 1970; 126: 1245–51.
11. In re *Quinlan, Supreme Court of New Jersey* 1976. 70 N.J.10,355A2d647, *certiori* denied 429 U.S.922, 97S. Ct.319, 50L.Ed.2d289 (1976).
12. Levine RJ. *Ethics and Regulation of Clinical Research*, 2nd ed. New Haven, CT: Yale University Press, 1988.

13. Fellner CH. Organ donation: For whose sake? *Ann Intern Med*, 1973; 79: 589–92.
14. Ad Hoc Committee at Harvard Medical School to Examine the Definition of Brain Death. A definition of irreversible coma. *JAMA*, 1968; 205: 337–40.
15. Sadler HH. The motivation of living donors. *Transplant Proc*, 1973; 5(2): 1121–3.
16. Advisory Committee to the Renal Transplant Registry. The ninth report of the Human Renal Transplant Registry. *JAMA*, 1972; 220(2): 253–60.
17. Rettig RA. Historical perspective. In: Levinsky NG, ed. *Ethics and the Kidney*. Oxford: Oxford University Press, 2001; 3–23.
18. Spital A. Evolution of attitudes at U.S. transplant centers toward kidney donation by friends and altruistic strangers. *Transplantation*, 2000; 69(8): 1728–31.
19. Humar A, Durand B, Gillingham K, Payne WD, Sutherland DE, Matas AJ. Living unrelated donors in kidney transplants: Better long-term results than with non-HLA-identical living related donors? *Transplantation*, 2000; 69(9): 1942–5.
20. Matas AJ, Garvey CA, Jacobs CL, Kahn JP. Nondirected donation of kidneys from living donors. *N Engl J Med*, 2000; 343(6): 433–6.
21. Crowley-Matoka M, Switzer G. Nondirected living donation: A survey of current trends and practices. *Transplantation*, 2005; 79(5): 515–9.
22. Adams PL, Cohen DJ, Danoovitch GM, *et al.* The nondirected live-kidney donor: Ethical considerations and practice guidelines: A National Conference Report. *Transplantation*, 2002; 74(4): 582–90.
23. Hilhorst MT, Kranenburg LW, Zuidema W, *et al.* Altruistic living kidney donation challenges: Psychosocial research and policy: A response to previous articles. *Transplantation*, 2005; 79(11): 1470–4.
24. Spital A. More on directed kidney donation by altruistic living strangers: A response to Dr. Hilhorst and his colleagues. *Transplantation*, 2005; 80(8): 1001–2.
25. Jacobs CL, Roman D, Garvey C, Kahn J, Matas AJ. Twenty-two nondirected kidney donors: An update on a single center's experience. *Am J Transplant*, 2004; 4: 1110–6.
26. Majors D. The gifted who keeps on giving. Post-gazette.com (the interactive edition of the *Pittsburgh Post-Gazette*). Available at http://www.post-gazette.com/printer.asp. July 23, 2003.

Part VII

The big picture: organizational issues

25

It's not my responsibility

Mary Beth Foglia and Robert A. Pearlman

Case narrative

As chair of the ethics committee, I (RAP) received a phone call from a second-year cardiology research fellow requesting advice about a vexing case. She asked the following question:

What are the ethical considerations in a case in which a resident moonlighting at a free-standing urgent-care clinic ignored the fellow's interpretation of an EKG showing an acute heart attack and treated a patient with shortness of breath for possible pneumonia? When the patient returned to the clinic the following day because of worsening symptoms, the resident sent the patient to the hospital without the initial EKG. The patient died shortly after admission.

I asked the fellow to tell me more about the case. She reported that a 68-year-old patient with a host of chronic medical problems including emphysema, diabetes, and congestive heart failure went to an urgent-care clinic for evaluation of increased difficulty in breathing. A moonlighting resident examined the patient and ordered an EKG, chest X-ray, and lab tests. The resident interpreted the EKG as clinically insignificant and thought that the chest X-ray showed findings consistent with the patient's emphysema. The resident also noted what appeared to be a possible infection behind the heart. Laboratory tests showed a mildly elevated white blood cell count, but no tests were ordered to rule out a heart attack. The resident diagnosed a possible pneumonia, prescribed antibiotics, and told the patient to return if his symptoms did not improve.

The resident, a trainee at a local medical center, worked in freestanding urgent-care clinics during off-hours with a business partner who was an internal medicine fellow. When the patient was initially examined the resident sent the EKG via facsimile to the business/home of the partner with a request for interpretation

The authors wish to thank Thomas Gallagher, MD, and Virginia Ashby Sharpe, PhD, for their helpful critique of this work.

("What's your impression of this EKG?"). The business partner and the fellow who requested the ethics consultation share a house together. The partner was not home, but the fellow saw the EKG and interpreted it as suggestive of an acute heart attack. She called the resident to report her findings, but he had already discharged the patient, telling the patient to return if his symptoms did not improve. The resident was not inclined to call the patient back to the clinic or to tell him to go to an emergency room (ER).

The patient returned the next day with worsening symptoms. The same resident arranged ambulance transport to the ER of an inner-city teaching hospital. The accompanying medical records did not include the initial EKG, the fellow's interpretation of the EKG, or any other information suggesting the patient was having a heart attack. The ER physicians thought that the patient had an exacerbation of his emphysema and admitted him to the hospital's medical unit. The fellow somehow knew that the patient was being admitted to the hospital's medical service and had him rerouted to the intensive-care unit (ICU). The fellow told the ICU staff about the patient's clinical presentation approximately 28 hours before, including the initial EKG. Treatment for an acute heart attack was begun. Despite intensive care, the patient's condition deteriorated and he died within a day of admission.

After hearing this case summary I reviewed it with my coethics consultant for the month. Good ethics starts with good facts. We agreed that we needed to further clarify the facts of the case before proceeding with the ethical analysis. We called the fellow back to clarify the goals of the consultation from her perspective. The fellow stated, "I want to understand the ethics of the case and hear options about how to respond." We then called the resident to learn more about his view of the case. We were especially interested in understanding why he decided not to notify the patient when he received the fellow's interpretation of the EKG and why he chose not to send the EKG with the patient to the ER. The resident refused to discuss the case with us and did not answer subsequent phone calls. Next we talked with a cardiology attending physician at our facility to ascertain the standards of practice in responding to an acute heart attack. The attending identified measures that significantly reduce the likelihood of death if implemented as soon as a heart attack is suspected. Therefore, *if* the patient was suffering an acute heart attack at the original clinic visit, the delay in treatment very likely contributed to his death. We also talked with the ICU attending physician (the unit where the patient died) to see if she would talk with the resident to learn more about what happened. She stated, "I do not and will not assume the role of an investigative cop." She reported that it was impossible to know if the care provided at the original clinic was causally related to the patient's death. Next we called the directors of the resident and fellows training programs at the university to explore their interest in and responsibility for the behavior of their trainees. Both directors said moonlighting is discouraged but not prohibited, that this behavior was outside their control, and that they did not want to get involved. Lastly, we communicated with our hospital's lawyers and were told the hospital was not liable for this outcome. The lawyers had no formal opinion about whether the deceased patient's family should be told of the possible link between his original care and his death. We did not contact the patient's wife or review the patient's medical record at this time.

Our next step was to schedule a meeting of the full ethics committee to explore how to respond to the case. Prior to this meeting, we concluded that the resident was most likely "covering up" his missteps in the care of this patient. I was outraged by this resident's apparent recklessness (i.e., knowing that an action or omission involves an unacceptable level of risk and taking the risk anyway) in concealing information material to the patient's care from our facility.[1] Even more disturbing, however, was the fact that the patient likely died as a result of these missteps and the patient's wife had no insight into this possibility. She was uninformed, powerless, and currently without recourse. We pressed ahead and asked the ethics committee to help us consider the following questions:

1. Should the state's medical board be contacted to conduct a formal, independent review of the case? And if so, whose responsibility should it be to inform the board?

2. Does our institution have a responsibility to communicate the suspicion of a serious medical error to the wife of the deceased patient to allow her to seek redress if she so chooses?

3. Is it appropriate for an ethics consultation service/ethics committee to assume a more direct advocacy role (e.g., contact the medical board and/or disclose to the wife directly) rather than a consultative role with regard to ensuring a just outcome in a case like this?

Haunting aspects

Even before meeting with the ethics committee I experienced a significant degree of moral distress. Three features of the case contributed to my disquiet. First, I always try to clarify the perspectives of stakeholders in an ethics case. Stakeholders are defined as those individuals (or groups) most likely to derive benefit or be harmed by institutional decisions.[2] Yet in this case I couldn't elicit the resident's first-person account because he was unwilling to talk with me. Second, because the requester (fellow) was not directly involved in the deceased patient's care I did not feel empowered to contact his family. Moreover, the intensive-care physician declined to get involved. I hoped she would serve as a proxy for my interest in seeing resolution to the ethical challenges posed by this case. Finally, I sensed that because the behavior in question occurred during off-hours, outside the walls of the hospital, and by nonhospital staff, no one in the medical center felt any responsibility to get involved.

My distress increased when the ethics committee met to discuss the case. The contentious committee process lasted for several hours over two days. One member of the committee who at first said we should not even discuss the case because it gets us involved later rose to his feet and said, "If you want to report this resident to the medical board, you do it. I do not want to be a party to this!" Although a consensus among committee members was ultimately achieved, it came at a price. We agreed to validate the fellow's moral intuition about the case, share the committee's deliberations, and focus our communication on the requester's questions and needs. Committee members agreed that not sending the original EKG to the inner-city hospital and concealing the possibility that the patient had suffered a heart attack appeared to be intentional departures from safe clinical practice standards[1] and an ethics violation. The committee felt that misinterpreting the EKG and disregarding the interpretation and advice of a cardiologist-in-training were problematic from a medical education or training perspective – an unintended medical error[1] – but were not necessarily moral errors.[3] The committee concluded that the fellow should be encouraged to report the case to the medical board if she believed, after deliberating about the ethical analysis, that the resident's behavior deserved formal, independent review. Committee members realized, however, that the fellow's personal entanglements would likely restrain her follow-up with the moonlighting resident. Additionally, we recognized that even experienced physicians are loathe to confront other physicians about their clinical practice.[4] I felt that our response (i.e., encourage the fellow to report the resident if she concurred with our analysis) was weak and ineffectual but probably appropriate all things considered.

As chair of the committee I felt we had just survived a battle involving the collision of disparate and strongly held personal convictions. The resultant wounds were only partially allayed by our agreed-upon outcome. Thus, I felt challenged to strategize how and when to debrief this case, both to ensure that we learned from our collective experience and to rebuild trust between committee members and a sense of integrity in the consultation process. In addition, I had yet to come to grips with my own deeply held and ongoing conviction that the patient's wife was unfairly excluded from the process and that she was not given an opportunity to seek redress or closure for the reported behavior and its possible link to her husband's death. I had the uneasy feeling that procedural justice (responding within an understood scope of practice for ethics consultants and achieving consensus among committee members) had come at the expense of achieving a just outcome for this patient's family.[5] Shklar, in her book *Faces of Injustice*, argues that we are passively unjust when we fail to ameliorate harm simply because it falls outside a system of justice rules. She believes that a conception of justice reducible to an adherence to a set of procedures is deeply impoverished – placing the interests of more powerful stakeholders ahead of the interests of less powerful stakeholders.[6] It is this nagging sense that we were "passively unjust" that makes it difficult for me to put this case to bed once and for all.

Ultimately, the committee concluded that it was not our role or responsibility as consultants to right a presumed wrong when the principals in the case resisted or refused to follow our recommendations (e.g., resident, fellow, ICU attending physician, training institution, etc.). Furthermore, we believed that acting as the "ethics police" (by reporting the resident to the medical board for possibly concealing an error) would inhibit future requests for consultation and undermine the value of our service. Thus, even as individuals we should not communicate our concerns to the state board of medicine. With a certain degree of hesitancy I came to the conclusion that although I (and we as a committee) had the power to make the situation (more) right, neither I nor the committee perceived that we had the authority. Our authority to act was constrained by the ethics facilitation role ascribed to ethics consultants within our facility – that is, our primary job as consultants is to identify and analyze value uncertainties and to facilitate consensus around ethically permissible courses of action[7] – recommending but not obligating or enforcing actions for others to take.

Professional reflections

This case occurred before the release of the landmark Institute of Medicine (IOM) report, "To Err is Human: Building a Safer Health Care Institution."[8] The IOM report paints a sobering portrait of a healthcare system where serious medical errors are ubiquitous and disclosure to patients is anomalous. The IOM report reinforced the goals of the patient-safety movement: to minimize preventable adverse events and to create a culture where medical error reporting and disclosure becomes the norm.[8] Achieving these goals depends on moving from a culture of secrecy and blame where errors are viewed as atypical events indicating personal failure to a culture where errors are regarded as the inescapable consequence of complex medical systems and as opportunities to improve patient safety.[9] The IOM report calls for greater transparency, establishing requirements for error reporting and obligations of full disclosure following harmful errors. This "duty to disclose" to patients or family has been codified by accrediting bodies,[10] state law,[11] and proposed action by Congress.

In retrospect, readers of this case may be right to observe that ethics committees are flawed, fallible, and sometimes shortsighted, offering recommendations that are not always prescient and that are delimited by our personal experiences, historic times, and the organizational context in which we serve. Thus, humility is a virtue to be cultivated – keeping us open to a re-examination of our decisions and actions in light of new insights. It is even fair to suggest that our committee was complicit with the prevailing "culture of silence" even as we agonized about the wife being kept in the dark about the circumstances surrounding her husband's death. Today we may have made a more muscular case supported by institutional policy and culture that disclosing to the patient's wife and ensuring an independent review of the resident's seemingly reckless behavior (i.e., not sending the original EKG and the fellow's interpretation of the EKG to the ER with the patient) was ethically obligatory – even if it required direct action by the ethics committee to ensure this outcome. Benjamin Freedman[12] argues that ethics consultants "must be prepared for the possibility of losing his or her job at any time over some action needed to protect the interests of patients." Therefore, some cases may require the moral courage to subordinate the interests of the ethics committee and its future activities to the interests of seeing justice served – especially because in most healthcare organizations there is no appeal to justice higher than the ethics committee. If we are unwilling to act, who is?

That being said, even if our committee's deliberations had resulted in an independent review of the resident's actions and disclosure to the decedent's wife, these outcomes would not have corrected the underlying systems issues that contributed to the patient's death. This requires an organizational or systems-level approach. Traditional, case-based ethics consultation results in solutions that may resolve the immediate case but do little to prevent a reoccurrence of the problem. The problem recurs because the underlying systems and processes that contribute causally to the problem remain unchanged.[13] In this case, contributory systems issues included a lack of systematic processes for identifying and addressing doctors whose performance poses a substantial threat to patients,[4] the training institution's policy toward moonlighting residents, a professional culture that shames and blames those who admit their mistakes, a lack of oversight of the resident's practice by a more senior clinician, and the lack of an institutional mechanism for addressing quality of care and ethical issues across healthcare organizations.

A systems perspective may not alter the case analysis or the conclusion reached by the ethics committee or consultant. However, a systems approach presumes that ethics cases are imbedded in and influenced by a larger organizational context – drawing attention to facets of the case that might otherwise have been overlooked or marginalized. Ethics consultants should always look "upstream" from their case for predisposing and contributory factors. Recurrent cases predict future cases unless the underlying systems-level antecedents are identified and addressed. An organizational or systems approach provides a means of preventing the reoccurrence of ethically indefensible outcomes.[13]

Outcome

My hospital's chief of staff oversees the ethics consultation service. As part of this oversight she reviewed our case analysis and sent a letter to the medical director of the freestanding urgent-care clinic (without copying the decedent's wife) suggesting that the case be reviewed due to the patient's death shortly following admission to the hospital. This is standard institutional policy when a patient is transferred to us from another care setting and dies within 24 hours of admission. No further follow-up occurred. We have no knowledge of what, if any action, the fellow took and presume that the wife remains unaware of the sequence of events that may have contributed to her husband's untimely death.

Discussion questions

1. What would you have done differently in this case? Why?
2. If this case had also been referred to an organizational ethics committee, how might the outcome have been different? Are there systems issues the ethics committee left unaddressed in this case that an organizational ethics committee might have been better equipped to resolve?
3. In your view, was the ethics committee obliged to ensure that the decedent's wife understood that the care received by her husband at the clinic might have contributed to his death?
4. The committee was concerned it would be perceived as the "ethics police" if it reported the resident to the medical board and that this would adversely affect clinicians' trust in the service and reduce future referrals. What do you think about this argument?
5. In your opinion, should ethics consultants ever move from a consultative/facilitation role to an advocacy role? If so, what criteria should ethics consultants/services use to make this decision?

REFERENCES

1. Merry A, McCall Smith A. *Errors, Medicine, and the Law.* Cambridge: Cambridge University Press, 2001.
2. Phillips R. *Stakeholder Theory and Organizational Ethics.* San Francisco: Berrett-Koehler Publishers, 2003.
3. Bosk CL. *Forgive and Forget: Managing Medical Failure.* Chicago: University of Chicago Press, 1979.
4. Leape LL, Fromson JA. Problem doctors: Is there a systems-level solution? *Ann Intern Med,* 2006; 144: 107–15.
5. Reitemeier PJ. Quality and error in bioethics consultation: A puzzle in pieces. In: Rubin SB, Zoloth L, eds. *Margin of Error: The Ethics of Mistakes in the Practice of Medicine.* Hagerstown, MD: University Publishing Group, 2000; 231–49.
6. Aulisio MP, Arnold RM, Younger SJ. *Ethics Consultation: From Theory to Practice.* Baltimore: Johns Hopkins University Press, 2003.
7. Kohn LT, Corrigan JM, Donaldson MS, eds. *To Err Is Human: Building a Safer Health Care System.* Washington, DC: National Academy Press, 1999.
8. Sharpe VA. *Accountability, Patient Safety and Policy Reform.* Washington, DC: Georgetown University Press, 2004.
9. Joint Commission on Accreditation of Healthcare Organizations. *Ethical Issues and Patient Rights Across the Continuum of Care.* Oakbrook Terrace, IL: Joint Commission on Accreditation of Healthcare Organizations Press, 1996.

10. Eads J. State mandates reporting of unusual incidents and medical errors. *Tenn Med*, 2002; 95(6): 239–40.

11. Freedman B. From avocation to vocation: Working conditions for clinical bioethicists. In: Baylis F, ed. *The Health Care Ethics Consultant*. Totawa, NJ: Humana Press, 1994; 109–32.

12. Foglia MB, Pearlman RA. Integrating clinical and organizational ethics: A systems perspective can provide an antidote to the "silo" problem in clinical ethics consultations. *Health Progr*, 2006; 87(2): 31–5.

13. Shklar JN. *The Faces of Injustice*. New Haven, CT: Yale University Press, 1990.

26

Intra-operative exposure to sporadic Creutzfeldt-Jakob disease: to disclose or not to disclose

Joel Potash

Case narrative

As senior ethics consultant on-call for the month, I received a telephone call from a hospital administrator requesting the opinion of the ethics committee prior to the department of health visiting the following day. The dilemma was whether a patient who may have been exposed to sporadic Creutzfeldt-Jakob disease (CJD) by surgical instruments during a brain operation should be informed of the exposure in view of the remote chance of the patient contracting CJD and the likely immediate and continuing emotional distress to the patient.

The patient, no longer in the hospital, had brain surgery 11 days before. The instruments used for the patient's operation were in one of six sets used on the day of the patient's operation. One of these sets had been used the previous day for a brain operation. The pathology report for that operation, which listed unsuspected CJD, did not arrive until all neurosurgical operations on the day of the patient's surgery had been completed. All operative instruments had undergone routine cleaning and sterilization, which may have been inadequate to kill the prions responsible for CJD. In fact, in the case of CJD the Centers for Disease Control and Prevention (CDC) recommends cleaning and sterilization techniques that are not generally used because they may be harmful to the surgical instruments or, alternatively, disposal of such instruments.

It is unusual to receive a request from hospital administration regarding a clinical case, especially regarding a patient already discharged and with the urgency occasioned by a department of health review. Although the request was for the opinion of the ethics committee, due to its urgency I established an ad hoc subcommittee consisting of myself and two other senior ethics consultants at the hospital to meet with the patient's neurosurgeon and neurologist. Prior to this meeting I read texts and journal articles about this uncommon disease and its rare potential for intraoperative neurosurgical transmission. CJD has an incidence of one to two cases per 1 million population. Sporadic CJD has been reported to be transmitted by contaminated neurosurgical instruments, corneal transplants, dura mater grafts, cadaveric pituitary growth hormone extract injections, and implanted brain electrodes.[1] The incubation time for iatrogenic CJD is 0.6 to 2.2 years.[1] Sporadic CJD prions have also been found in spleen, muscles, and olfactory tissues.[2]

I spoke with physicians in infectious diseases involved with this case. The neurosurgeon provided a personal communication from the CDC listing six likely cases of CJD linked to exposure to contaminated neurosurgical instruments. Three occurred in the 1950s and one in 1980, but two more recent cases were difficult to assess due to hospital closings and unavailability of medical records. The communication, later published, stated: "The absence of recent CJD cases associated with neurosurgical procedures was believed to be due to advances in standard hospital sterilization procedures . . . In a minority of these incidents personnel made a decision to inform patients exposed to neurosurgical instruments that were not cleaned using the recommended CJD decontamination methods."[3]

At the ad hoc committee meeting, the patient's neurologist and the neurosurgeon expressed concern about the patient's reaction to disclosure of this event, given that the patient had been emotionally distraught about the lack of control of her neurological disease and put all her hopes on a successful surgical outcome.

The ad hoc committee first discussed the reasons in favor of disclosure to the patient of possible exposure to sporadic CJD:

1. Respect for the autonomy of patients demands that they be given information relative to their health, or in this case to their future health, unless they refuse such information. While the odds of the procedure causing CJD in this patient are remote, if CJD occurs it is invariably fatal and associated with considerable suffering. However, at the present time there is no diagnostic test for CJD except biopsy of the brain, and there is no treatment available.
2. Our state grants patients access to their medical records. Patients often authorize release of their medical records to their healthcare providers. If the possible exposure is mentioned in medical records or communication, the patient may learn of it, leading to lack of trust in the physicians and hospital involved.
3. In the future, presymptomatic diagnosis and treatment of CJD may become available. Patients would need to know of their exposure to access these.
4. Should the patient develop CJD, even though it was unintended and unavoidable, the patient might be deserving of compensation.
5. Without knowledge of exposure to CJD, the patient might ignore neurological symptoms and not seek timely medical attention.
6. While there would be no changes in the patient's lifestyle due to possible CJD exposure, she would not be allowed to donate blood, corneas, or other tissues. She would also not be allowed to be an anatomical donor.
7. Other patients would be at risk if this patient were to leave her physicians or geographic area and require further brain surgery.

Reasons supporting nondisclosure are as follows:
1. The principle of therapeutic privilege allows a physician to withhold information from a patient if disclosure would cause the patient significant emotional distress.
2. There is only a one-in-six chance that this patient has been exposed, and even exposure may not lead to CJD.
3. There is no treatment for CJD, so the course of the disease would not be changed.
4. There appears to be nothing that needs to be done to protect others even if the patient develops CJD, unless she undergoes further neurosurgery.

The ad hoc committee considered that on balance, weighing potential harms and benefits to the patients and others, the patient should be informed of the possible risk to her of acquiring CJD. The patient has a right to this information, and the physician has a duty to disclose the circumstances leading to the risk, including the low likelihood of acquiring CJD, in a compassionate and supportive way. The physician and the hospital should offer psychological counseling, if desired, at no expense to the patient. It is reasonable to delay disclosure until the patient's neurologist feels the patient is best able to deal with it emotionally. Both physicians involved should be present at disclosure as well as any family members or others the patient invites. The physicians might wish to make other medical personnel expert in CJD and its transmission available to the patient and her family. Respect for the patient's confidentiality allows disclosure only to those whom the patient has authorized to receive information; confidentiality should not be overridden in this case, especially since others are not at apparent risk. The patient needs to be advised about the possible harms of self-disclosure. We stated that if the patient's physicians decided disclosure was not appropriate, we would want to meet with them again for further discussion. Hospital counsel was already aware of this case.

The DOH concluded that a neurosurgical instrument used in the biopsy of the patient with CJD was used the following day for our patient's brain operation. The instrument was used after routine sterilization, which may be inadequate for contamination with CJD. The DOH recommended that the hospital ensure the ethics committee addresses patient notification concerning the safety of blood supply should the patient donate blood. It also recommended the hospital address prevention of exposure to others if the patient undergoes subsequent brain surgery.

I contacted the regional medical director of the American Red Cross and learned that the Food and Drug Administration prohibited blood donation from anyone at risk for CJD. The regional Red Cross had an additional policy of not accepting blood donors who were recipients of cadaveric corneal transplants or cadaveric human pituitary extract injections for fear of transmitting CJD. Prohibitions against donors in these categories are lifelong. If a blood donor is later found to have CJD, the regional Red Cross recommends that the recipient patients be notified of this. I also discussed the case with the head of risk management and later with hospital counsel.

I again met with the neurosurgeon involved and discussed the certainty that she used an instrument that had undergone standard sterilization after being used for a brain operation on a patient with CJD. Although the neurosurgeon's department chair recommended patient notification of the potential risk of CJD, the neurosurgeon was undecided as to whether she would notify the patient. I emphasized even more strongly that the patient has a right to know the risk of CJD, even if it is very small, and what it means regarding blood, tissue, or organ donation. We also discussed what it may mean to others if the patient requires further brain surgery. I believed that compassion and care in communicating the information could minimize the patient's emotional suffering.

Haunting aspects

In this case I weighed the likelihood of causing the patient immediate and possibly enduring emotional harm against the unlikely future harm of CJD. There is currently no treatment for CJD, which is invariably fatal.

A troubling aspect was the request for an ethics consultation by hospital administration in the face of a DOH review after the patient had left the hospital. The DOH review charged the ethics committee with addressing the safety of blood supply and surgical instruments. The neurosurgeon, not the ethics consultant, is an expert on these topics, and I expected her to be responsible for them. Hospital administration was concerned at first with whether disclosure was indicated with this particular patient. Later, the DOH added the concern for the well-being of other patients and the general public if this patient donated blood or organs in the future. I had no opportunity to meet with the patient to assess whether the "therapeutic privilege" of physician nondisclosure was applicable, but a psychiatric consultation would accomplish that better.

My report was sent to administration. I was not sure whether it would find its way into an inpatient or ambulatory chart for later reference. I copied the patient's neurosurgeon with my consultation note. I couldn't see how the patient's physicians could discuss contraindication to blood donation (whether scientifically valid or not) and organ donation and concerns about future surgeries without discussing the patient's possible iatrogenic exposure during her neurosurgery and its potential effects.

As an ethics consultant, I have occasionally discussed my concerns about other ethics consultations with medical directors, hospital attorneys, and administrators. I remind myself that a medical consultant merely offers recommendations to the requesting physicians, who may accept or reject them. I have no authority other than moral suasion to effect my recommendations. In other ethics consultations I occasionally found no indication in the medical chart that my consultation note had been read or its recommendations followed. I am often not copied on discharge summaries, but our consultation team proactively acquires discharge summaries for all inpatients on whom we consult. On several occasions I asked the administrator who requested the original consultation about whether this patient had been told of her risk and never received the promised response. I asked risk management whether disclosure had been made and also received no reply. I approached the neurosurgeon periodically and was told that the patient had not yet been told but would be. I was unsure whose anxiety we were dealing with, the patient's or the physician's. I feel a need to be more proactive in the future to discover how my consultations effect solutions to moral dilemmas that are presented to me in requests for ethics consultations. However, I do not want to be considered the "ethics policeman" because that may avert future consultations.

Professional reflections

While I respect patients' rights to refuse information, I wonder whether they can make good decisions about difficult choices without sufficient knowledge. However, "sufficient" knowledge varies from patient to patient: not too much and not too little, as much as the patient needs, as much as the patient wants, what the physician usually tells. In the case of this patient, determining what she would want to know seemed impossible without revealing the prospect, albeit miniscule, of an iatrogenic, untreatable, and always fatal disease. There seemed to be three possible approaches: (a) tell the patient now or in the near future, (b) never tell the patient and hope that she does not get CJD, and (c) delay telling the patient until after the usual period of incubation for neurosurgically acquired CJD of 6–22 months. I believed the first case to be the right choice and the second to be a wrong choice. Disclosure beyond the incubation period, a less desirable alternative, may result in the patient responding with relief and gratitude or anger and loss of trust in the physician and the hospital. I worried about losing track of the patient if she moved away without notifying her physicians. I was concerned about the patient having access to future presymptomatic diagnostic testing or research trials of treatment for CJD. I believed that if she developed CJD, she should be compensated for her iatrogenic disease if she desired. She might not be if she did not know of her exposure. I worried that other people would be exposed to neurosurgical instruments used on the patient if she needed further brain surgery at another hospital. I wanted to ensure that the patient never let her health insurance lapse in case she came down with CJD and was then uninsurable.

These concerns bothered me even though I understood that the odds were against the patient contracting CJD, and they outweighed my concern for the emotional distress the patient would likely experience if her risk were disclosed. I know of patients with family histories of Huntington's disease (HD) who have refused to be tested for HD because they did not want to learn whether they had an untreatable disease and because the knowledge of having HD would likely cause them to be emotionally distraught for many presymptomatic years. The risk to our patient of contracting CJD was much less. A patient with HD might need to make decisions about pregnancy or prenatal testing. Our patient would not have to make any changes in lifestyle other than those regarding blood, organ, and body donation. There seemed to be no way to know which side of the disclosure argument this patient would be on. In a similar quandary involving the recipient of blood from a donor who later died of variant CJD (mad cow disease), Steinberg concluded that the recipient should be notified, although he found a decision to withhold information morally defensible.[4] I too felt the patient should be told, but I found the decision not to disclose more difficult to defend.

As consultants we ought to remind physicians continually of the limitations of paternalism and therapeutic privilege. Most patients want to know about their health problems. Physicians cannot protect patients from all suffering, but they can modify suffering with compassion and continuing care. Ethics consultants have little power to force disclosure in a case like this other than through moral suasion. It is important for physicians to develop a habit of truthful disclosure and to display the courage needed to discuss bad news with their patients. Bending the truth or avoiding disclosure in a case like this may make it easier to do the same in other, less unusual cases.

Outcome

After recovering from neurosurgery, the patient's neurosurgeon and neurologist recommended that the patient avoid blood or organ donation in view of her medical problems. They did not mention the risk of developing CJD. The patient expressed no inclination to donate blood or organs in the future. This satisfied the DOH's concern of protecting the public. The patient was observed for indications of CJD. More than two years after her surgery the physicians told the patient of possible intraoperative exposure to CJD. She expressed acceptance but not gratitude, anger, or emotional distress. She refused an offer to discuss her situation with a physician expert in CJD. Since this case occurred, there have been several cases of variant CJD from blood transfusion but no cases of sporadic CJD from blood transfusion. The Red Cross still does not accept blood from anyone at risk for CJD, nor do organ donation centers accept organs from persons potentially exposed to CJD. Accepting anatomical gifts of bodies from patients with CJD or at risk for CJD is strongly discouraged.

We ethics consultants and the ethics committee did not recommend changes in hospital policy regarding therapeutic privilege. While it is a relief to me that the patient was finally informed of her iatrogenic risk for CJD, her lack of emotional response does not seem to support her physician's initial reasoning against early disclosure. The patient's response does not seem to contribute much to either side of the argument, and the literature involving the few cases of transmission of CJD intraoperatively is not helpful. In cases like this one I will continue to recommend disclosure as the most respectful approach to the patient. I will continue to emphasize that bad news cannot be avoided in such situations, but it can be softened by the physician's compassion and nonabandonment. Belay states: "The circumstances surrounding such episodes vary and are best handled by a local hospital review board consisting of pertinent physicians, ethicists, hospital administrators, infection control professionals, and possibly others."[3] It would help me and other ethics consultants to learn the outcome of such deliberations, and I encourage the publication of such deliberations in medical literature.

Discussion questions

1. When access to the patient or a surrogate is not available, how can the ethics consultant assess the patient's concerns regarding an ethical dilemma? Should the consultation proceed under such circumstances?
2. Because the request for consultation came from hospital administration, should the consultant ask that the consultation notes forwarded to hospital administration be included in the patient's hospital record as a postscript? Should ethics consultants' notes always be entered directly in medical charts?
3. What power, if any, do ethics consultants and the ethics committee have to force the patient's physician to comply with their recommendation to disclose? May the ethics consultants report the physician's inaction to the hospital administration, the department of health, or the state office of professional misconduct, particularly given the mandate of the DOH in this case?

REFERENCES

1. Johnson RT, Gibbs CJ Jr. Creutzfeldt-Jakob Disease and related transmissible spongiform encephalopathies. *N Engl J Med*, 1998; 339(27): 1998–9.
2. Glatzel M, Abela E, Maissen M, Aguzzi A. Extraneural pathologic prion protein in sporadic Creutzfeldt-Jakob Disease. *N Engl J Med*, 2003; 349(19): 1812.
3. Belay ED, Schonberger LB. The public health impact of prion disease. *Annu Rev Publ Health*, 2005; 26: 195.
4. Steinberg D. Informing a recipient of blood from a donor who developed Creutzfeldt-Jakob Disease: The characteristics of information that warrant its disclosure. *J Clin Ethics*, 2001; Summer: 136.

27

Why do we have to discharge this patient?

Sarah E. Shannon

Case narrative

At this medium-sized urban hospital, the chair of the ethics committee usually responded to requests for ethics consultations by either personally doing consults, referring others to another member of the committee who was either on-call or knowledgeable about a specific issue, or by convening the entire ethics committee to discuss challenging cases. I was a community member, recruited by the chair due to my academic appointment and credentials in ethics. I received a phone call over the weekend that there would be an urgent ethics committee meeting on Tuesday morning at 7 a.m. An ethics consultation request had been received on Friday. The ethics committee chair had reviewed the case and decided it merited full committee review.

Approximately ten clinicians and other hospital employees were present for the Tuesday morning meeting. We learned immediately that Mr. Leary, the patient, had died the evening before at his home. The rest of the case unfolded in the ensuing discussion. Mr. Leary was described as an independent 76-year-old curmudgeon prior to a stroke eight weeks ago. The stroke left him with complete left-sided paralysis. He suffered a second stroke two weeks after the first, resulting in both receptive and expressive aphasia – he could neither understand speech nor could he formulate words. He also appeared depressed after the second event. Three weeks ago, he suffered a third stroke. While this stroke worsened his physical condition, it seemed to improve his mood. At times, he appeared almost jovial. He became cooperative with care, even attempting to assist with shaving each morning.

Mr. Leary needed a feeding tube for nutrition and hydration since the first stroke due to an impaired swallow reflex. He tolerated a nasogastric feeding tube and had never attempted to remove the tube. His physician had written in the medical record that Mr. Leary's prognosis for survival was probably less than a year due to expected further cerebral events but that he might live as long as three to five years.

The clinicians who knew Mrs. Leary described her as overwhelmed with her husband's situation. In the eight weeks of hospitalization since Mr. Leary's first stroke, she had occasionally agreed to a "no-code" order when his condition was grim but would ask that he be restored to a full code when he improved. These changes appeared to follow discussions between the attending physician and Mrs. Leary but were never documented. In the last two weeks, Mr. Leary's condition had finally stabilized to the point where he could be discharged to a nursing home. The social worker had located two possible placements, but Mrs. Leary refused both. The first had been a 75-minute drive from her home, making visits difficult, and she had described the second as "too awful."

Late Thursday, someone from the hospital business office approached Mrs. Leary to inform her that on Monday Mr. Leary would be decertified by Medicare because he no longer required acute care and two nursing home placements had been offered. Since Mrs. Leary had refused transfer she would be responsible for hospital charges from that date forward. In line with hospital policy, no notation of this conversation was made in the medical record, but the nurses on the floor overheard the conversation. On Friday afternoon, Mrs. Leary called the attending physician and asked that the feeding tube be withdrawn, which they had discussed on other occasions but which Mrs. Leary had previously refused. She said that she had decided to take Mr. Leary home and care for him herself. The physician phoned the unit and left verbal orders to remove the feeding tube, discontinue nutrition and hydration, and discharge Mr. Leary to home as soon as feasible.

The nursing staff was very upset by the order to stop tube feeding and called the physician back to discuss it. He stated, "This is congruent with the patient's stated values prior to his strokes. The patient asked me not to 'overdo' it." The feeding tube was pulled Friday afternoon. The nurses remained distraught over the weekend and consulted the hospital chaplain, also a member of the ethics committee. They complained that while this physician spent a good deal of time with his patients and their families, he did not document conversations in the medical record and was curt with nursing staff when they tried to discuss patient or family issues. They felt silenced by him.

A social worker was not available over the weekend to help with discharge planning, but basic arrangements were made for the patient to be sent home Monday. On Sunday morning, the patient took a drink from a glass of water placed at his bedside for mouth care and aspirated water into his lungs. By Monday pneumonia was evident. Mrs. Leary was nearly hysterical. She had not participated actively in her husband's care and the nurses realized she was physically unable to turn and position Mr. Leary because of her diminutive size. Nonetheless, Mr. Leary was discharged home Monday afternoon with a significant fever. He died late Monday evening.

As details of the case were discussed in committee, many of the players saw their roles in a new light. The person from the business office was horrified when she realized the impact of her conversation on the patient's wife. She explained that Medicare regulations limited the number of times patients and families could reject transfers to nursing homes, but her words trailed off into silent tears. The patient's attending physician, an experienced clinician, had listened first with confidence. But when he learned about Mrs. Leary's conversation with the business office on Thursday he visibly blanched. He had not questioned Mrs. Leary's request to stop tube feeding because he felt she had been overly aggressive in her treatment preferences and assumed she had finally "seen reason." He spoke of the patient, clearly identifying with him on a personal level, and restated that he had promised the patient he would "not overdo it."

The oncologist gently questioned the attending physician about treatment of symptoms related to withdrawal of nutrition and hydration. The attending physician replied that the patient did not have pain so nothing was ordered. A discussion ensued about the duty to treat hunger, thirst, and anxiety related to withdrawal of life-sustaining treatments. The oncologist suggested that the patient's obvious symptoms of thirst should have been treated with good mouth care (as was done) and with medication. Next, the oncologist asked why the patient was being discharged at all. He pointed out that once the decision was made to withdraw tube feeding the patient's condition changed and he would have been recertified for Medicare reimbursement. Silence pervaded the room while everyone absorbed this crucial fact, somehow missed. Disbelief and horror were palpable in the room.

The social worker talked about her struggle to find placement during a period of high demand for nursing home beds. She was frustrated by recent budget cuts that limited social work coverage on the weekend, even for urgent discharge planning. She supported Mrs. Leary's refusal of the first nursing home because Mrs. Leary would not have been able to visit daily. The social worker was reluctant but obligated to offer the second placement, saying "I wouldn't put my dog in that place!"

Throughout the discussion, the nurses did not speak. They sat together, arms crossed, and directed hostile glances to the attending physician every time he spoke. Questions posed to the nurses were answered with terse replies. Their anger was palpable. When they realized that the attending physician had not known that losing Medicare reimbursement may have influenced the wife's decision, the nurses looked disbelieving, then distrustful. They repeated that Mr. Leary would assist them when they shaved him each morning, that he had never tried to remove his feeding tube, and that he laughed and had seemed happy the last two weeks. They had never heard him speak, so they had never heard him say he did not want tube feeding. They commented that the attending physician's notes were brief to the point of being cryptic. They said that what had happened to Mr. Leary was "wrong, simply wrong." They could not adequately provide discharge support over the weekend without social work assistance. Mr. Leary was dying when he was sent home; Mrs. Leary was in crisis. Though they did not say it, they appeared to blame the attending physician principally for these failures. But they also felt profound guilt. They had removed the tube. They had left the cup of water by the bedside. They helped put him on the stretcher, sick with fever, to go home with his wife to die. They had failed Mr. Leary.

The hospital administrator who attended the meeting sat silently through the discussion until the end. Then he spoke. "This isn't what we do. We don't abandon people. If we needed to eat a few days or even a week of care in order to adequately do discharge planning or to find a nursing home placement, then we would do that. But we don't abandon people." A policy decision was made on the spot. In the future, if a patient were being decertified for Medicare reimbursement, the physician would be notified prior to the patient or family being informed by the business office.

Haunting aspects

This case stands out for me as an example of ethics failure. First, this was a genuinely difficult case that needed careful ethical analysis. But the full consultation occurred too late to benefit the parties intimately involved in the case: most important, the patient. This highlights the second and perhaps most serious failure. The ethics consultation process failed to stop the train. The ethics consult was initiated on Friday. Yet, it failed to identify this as a situation that needed to be slowed down for careful reflection. The ethics consultant did not recommend that the level of care continue until careful reflection could occur. The consultant should have recommended that the feeding tube be left in place or replaced, whatever was necessary until the case could be discussed at the Tuesday morning meeting.

The third failure is that the ethics committee, upon realizing at the Tuesday meeting that a tragedy had occurred, failed to take action to help the many who were wounded by this case: the nurses who had correctly sensed that the situation presented authentic ethical issues yet continued to "follow orders" because they could not see other options; the social worker who felt personally responsible for not finding an adequate nursing home placement and frustrated to have not been at work during Mrs. Leary's acute discharge planning needs; the woman from the business office who was emotionally devastated and felt a distinct moral culpability for Mr. Leary's death; the attending physician who thought he had a sound clinical plan only to discover that several key facts were incorrect and that he had failed his longtime patient; and, of course, Mrs. Leary, who was now home alone, having spent the final ten hours of her husband's life frantically trying to care for his feverish and dying body alone and unaided. We, as a committee, did nothing about any of the wounded beyond our case discussion. Perhaps this was because we were overwhelmed or shamed by our own failure, or because we had not matured to a point where we could envision our role as providing solace for traumatized colleagues. Perhaps we were humbled by the complexities of this case, particularly the regulatory issues. Perhaps we responded like clinicians confronting medical errors by not fully admitting the error, not discussing it openly, and then not disclosing it to the affected parties.[1]

Professional reflections

There are four unique aspects to this case that continue to influence my practice in ethics consultation. The first was illustrated by the nurses' plaintive observations that although Mr. Leary could not understand verbal communication, he would cooperate with shaving each morning, turning his head from side to side, flattening his upper lip, and trying to hold the razor. He had not attempted to pull his feeding tube. And recently, he had seemed content, even laughing at times with the nurses as they cared for him. I came to understand that while the attending physician referenced prior verbal statements as indication of Mr. Leary's wishes, the nurses were reflecting on his current behavioral cues. Since it is not unusual for patients in Mr. Leary's condition to be withdrawn and rejecting, pushing away a helping hand and pulling out tubes, Mr. Leary's behavioral cues suggested to them that he accepted his situation and found meaning and contentment in life. We do not know how Mrs. Leary saw her husband's situation or how she weighed his prior verbal preferences against his current behavioral cues. Would his "former" self have judged his current quality of life unacceptable? Did his "current" self agree with that judgment? Perhaps she had no more insight into Mr. Leary's wishes than the nurses who shaved him each day and laughed with him about putting his slippers on the wrong feet.

One study of quality of life for nursing home residents found that physicians, family members, nurses, and certified nursing assistants (CNAs) rated the importance of quality of life similarly but rated their ability to influence residents' quality of life differently.[2] CNAs rated their ability to influence the quality of life of nursing home residents highest, while physicians rated theirs lowest. One explanation may be that the kind of patient care provided may carry with it a set of beliefs about the value that care has on the patient's quality of life. In this case, providing the intimate care of shaving, bathing, and dressing may have sensitized the nurses to the patient's nonverbal cues.

How can we as ethics consultants adjudicate between verbal or written preferences made by a "prior" self and the behavioral cues of the "current" self? When people can no longer speak, do their actions give voice to their wishes? Or, do their former voices shout while their current tears or smiles merely whisper? How should ethics consultants consider advance directives in light of these behavioral whispers?[3] I am unsure whether stopping nutrition and hydration was the best decision for Mr. Leary. The lack of discussion about his prior verbal statements balanced against his current behavioral cues denied him the opportunity to have these multiple voices heard.

The second lesson from this case was the power of interprofessional representation in ethics consultation. This was a complex case involving Medicare reimbursement, symptom management, neurological assessment, surrogate decision making, autonomy, and withholding life-sustaining nutrition and hydration. Interprofessional meetings bring expertise that allows multiple insights, questions, and possible solutions to emerge. This case also illustrates how ethics runs through an organization – from the business office through the service delivery groups to the administration. Representatives from each facet of the organization saw their role in this tragedy – from the business office person who delivered the news about decertification to the head of administration who would have gladly absorbed the cost of Mr. Leary's care for a limited time to avoid abandoning him. In ethics consultations, I have become more attuned to the need to gather information from multiple professionals and to have wide representation in case discussions.

The third lesson was the potential role of the ethics consultant in guiding clinicians toward moral certainty and courage. In retrospect, I believe that the ethics committee/consultant failed the nurses in this regard. The nurses requested the consultation. They recognized that something was not right. They also made mistakes. They did not tell the attending physician that the business office had visited Mrs. Leary because they assumed he knew. They did not try to talk further with the physician. They were angry with him and considered this to be the "final straw." They came to the ethics committee with their minds made up, perhaps hoping to see the attending physician publicly humiliated. Instead, they saw their own culpability. They stopped communicating with the physician, and in so doing failed their patient.

And where was the ethics consultant in this? Given what was known on Friday afternoon, we should have called the attending to share our recommendation to delay discontinuation of the tube feeding until after the interdisciplinary case discussion. If necessary, we should have supported the nurses in respectfully refusing to stop tube feeding until the discussion could occur. The ethics consultant could have spearheaded the process of contacting administration to clarify discharge and reimbursement issues. The alternative was unacceptable. Ethics consultants should see their role as guiding clinicians through situations where a clear stance and recommendation is warranted as a precursor to a final treatment decision. By demonstrating clear reasoning and a commitment to investigate the many dimensions of a complex case, the ethics consultant can support the clinicians in gaining clarity and taking a moral position.

Outcome

Within ten hours of being discharged home, with a fever, and in the sole care of his terrified and unprepared wife, Mr. Leary died. The ethics case discussion was too late and guilt for his death likely haunts the care providers, his wife, and ethics committee members to this day. I have used this case frequently and successfully in my teaching. While it is an excellent teaching tool, I use the case also to process my own guilt and to prevent other "Mr. and Mrs. Learys" from being abandoned.

Discussion questions

1. What are the ethics committee's obligations to the patient, his wife, the health-care professionals, and the organization?
2. How can an ethics consultant or committee ensure that relevant facts to the case emerge in a timely way? How do we ensure this even when we are not immediately aware of all the dimensions worthy of exploration?
3. How should an ethics committee help an organization heal and change after a case such as this? Should the ethics committee take leadership to heal the "wounded" or identify organizational change to prevent future tragedies?

REFERENCES

1. Hilfiker D. Facing our mistakes. *N Engl J Med*, 1984; 310(2): 118–22.
2. Kane RL, Rockwood T, Hyer K, *et al.* Rating the importance of nursing home residents' quality of life. *J Am Geriatr Soc*, 2005; 53(12): 2076–82.
3. Dresser R, Astrow AB. An alert and incompetent self: The irrelevance of advance directives. *Hastings Cent Rep*, 1998; 28(1): 28–30.

28

Who's that sleeping in my bed?
An institutional response to an
organizational ethics problem

Daryl Pullman, Rick Singleton, and Janet Templeton

Case narrative

Mr. Wiggins, 78, was admitted to our hospital for treatment of a stroke. His deficits included complete left-side weakness and slurred speech. His cognitive status was mildly impaired and he became frustrated and aggressive at times when unable to perform various activities. Indeed, Mr. Wiggins was dependent for all daily living activities, including hygiene and toileting. Although he completed his acute care and a period of convalescence, he did not regain any function on his left side.

Mr. Wiggins had maintained a very active lifestyle prior to the stroke. He and his wife of 53 years had lived together in their two-story home for over 40 years. Subsequent to the stroke and in consultation with the healthcare team, Mr. Wiggins and his family determined it would not be possible for him to return home. The family applied for placement in a nursing home. Per our institutional policy at the time, Mr. Wiggins and the family were invited to provide the names of three nursing homes. They selected St. Peter's as their first choice because this home was operated by their religious denomination. They also provided two other names.

After a three-month wait in acute care, a bed became available in one of the homes on the Wiggins family's list. However, it was not at St. Peter's, and the family subsequently declined this bed. Mr. Wiggins remained in acute care for an additional six months until a bed became available in their home of choice. In total, Mr. Wiggins remained in an acute-care bed for nine months after he was considered ready for medical discharge.

Cases like Mr. Wiggins were common in our hospital prior to the implementation of our "First Available Bed" policy. In some cases patients would occupy an acute-care bed for up to 18 months before a long-term care bed became available in their preferred institution. On average there were 43 patients waiting daily for transfer to a long-term care facility, and the average length of stay in acute care after medical discharge was 54 days. This situation was a continuing source of moral distress for managers of our acute-care units because it often resulted in the cancellation or postponement of acute-care services such as elective surgery or chemotherapy.

Few people plan to spend their final years in a long-term care facility. For many the decision to enter a nursing home comes at the end of an extended period of slow decline as it becomes increasingly clear they can no longer manage on their own. For others, like Mr. Wiggins, some catastrophic event necessitates the move. Irrespective of the proximate or final cause of the decision in favor of placement, it is often a decision of last resort for both the patient and family.[1] Emotions of grief, anger, helplessness, and remorse are often part and parcel of the process for all involved.[2] So prevalent are such negative emotions that "relocation stress syndrome" is now a recognized nursing diagnosis.[3] Numerous studies report that the stress of relocation can be ameliorated to some degree if the elderly patient is involved in the decision-making process and in the selection of a long-term care home.[4]

Professional reflections

There is an old adage in legal circles that states "tough cases make bad laws." It captures the wisdom that policy should not be based on exceptional cases. Societal laws and institutional policies must accommodate the vast majority of situations that arise in everyday life. If policies are set to respond to the exceptional case then the exception becomes the rule and the ordinary is made to conform to an extraordinary standard. For this reason the exceptional cases that haunt us in clinical practice often teach us much about the process of managing complex ethical problems, but they should generally not be used as guides when establishing institutional policies.

Ordinary cases like that of Mr. Wiggins, on the other hand, are generally not addressed through an ethics consultation service. Such cases occur on a somewhat regular basis in any institutional setting. While each is unique inasmuch as the individuals whose lives are captured in these events are unique, they do not make it onto the radar screen of the ethics consultation service. Nevertheless, as a class such cases lead to moral distress because they point to systemic inefficiencies in the management of a particular type of case. When such inefficiencies are identified within an organization the introduction of a new policy or procedure is an appropriate management strategy.

In Canada, stroke patients like Mr. Wiggins spend on average twice as many days in acute care as stroke patients in many other parts of the world.[5] The reasons for this are complex and include the fact that hospital care in Canada is funded entirely under provincial government health insurance plans, whereas nursing home care is only partially subsidized. However, acute-care units are not equipped to meet the ongoing needs of chronic-care patients. Recent research indicates that many elderly patients experience functional decline following acute-care hospital admissions. Extended stays can result in changes to cognitive as well as physical health.[6] Thus elderly patients who remain in acute-care beds beyond the time of medical discharge often receive suboptimal care. To deal with the ever-expanding problem of acute-care beds occupied by patients more appropriately placed elsewhere, many hospitals, regional health boards, and in some cases provinces in Canada have implemented "First Available Bed" policies in recent years.

After extensive consultation with regional partners our hospital decided to examine the merits of a "First Available Bed" policy. At that time our regional partners included the local nursing home board and the health and community services board. As the only tertiary-care facility in our region any change in hospital policy would affect these agencies directly. Our response included consultation with our organization's administrative ethics committee. This committee's mandate includes examining existing and proposed policies that could adversely affect patients or staff or that might otherwise undermine the organization's ability to accomplish its goals in an effective and efficient manner. Administrative ethics review tries to ensure that existing or prospective programs and policies are consistent with our organization's five core corporate values of respect for persons, caring community, justice and fairness, collaboration, and the pursuit of excellence.

When satisfied we had identified and addressed key ethical tensions between our responsibility to provide the best available care for individual patients and our duty to utilize limited healthcare resources in a fair and equitable manner, we moved to implement a "First Available Bed" policy. This policy requires that patients who are eligible for discharge from acute care complete an application for long-term care, which is submitted to a single-entry process. Although the patient is still permitted to identify a home of choice, when medically discharged the patient is transferred to the first available bed in the region that meets his or her assessed-care needs. Once transferred, the patient waits in long-term care for an internal transfer to the home of first choice. Following implementation of the policy the number of medically discharged patients waiting in acute care for transfer to a long-term care facility decreased from an average of 43 to 8 patients daily, and the average length of stay in acute care dropped from 54 to 10 days once the decision to apply for long-term care had been made.

Any institutional policy that affects patient care must be designed to alleviate institutional stress and to provide the best care for the patient. Hence we do not agree with those institutions that have developed a "First Available Bed" policy only as a contingency plan in crisis situations. When this occurs affected individuals may perceive the implementation as reactive rather than as a planned and principled means by which to provide appropriate care for patients who are medically discharged. If the justification for the policy is that it provides the most appropriate care for all patients, then it must be the most appropriate care irrespective of the availability of acute-care beds at any given time.

Haunting aspects

Our moral dilemma involves a clash between the principle of justice for all and the individual patient's autonomy rights. How do we strike an appropriate balance between the good of the whole and the rights of the individual patient? Viewed from the administrative distance afforded by statistical analysis of "average number of patients awaiting transfer" and "average length of stay in acute care after medical discharge," the "First Available Bed" policy is a clear success. Viewed from the perspective of individual patients and their families, however, the policy may appear insensitive at best and inhumane at worst. Indeed, despite our best efforts to implement our policy in a fair and equitable manner, our sense is that the majority of patients and families have come to tolerate this policy and process even though they are not in agreement with it.

Critics of "First Available Bed" policies argue that they discriminate on the basis of age and disability and that individual seniors are forced to bear the burden of an underfunded healthcare system and an underserviced community support program.[7] However, the force of such criticisms is mitigated when one shifts the moral lens away from those patients who currently occupy acute-care beds and who resent or resist efforts to move. The focus instead is on individuals who are deemed medically eligible for acute-care services but who must delay a necessary surgery or other medical intervention because the beds are otherwise occupied. Given the reality of limited healthcare resources and the general need to distribute what is available in a fair and equitable manner, the needs of patients who require acute-care beds because of their medical conditions would, all things considered, trump the preferences of those who are no longer medically eligible but who prefer not to move. Unfortunately the vast majority of patients in the latter category are seniors, but the fact that most of those affected by a policy fall into a certain demographic is insufficient grounds to claim the policy is *ipso facto* discriminatory.

Despite the in-principle support that can be garnered for a "First Available Bed" policy, in practice, there will be times when the policy is implemented in a ham-fisted fashion with predictably tragic results. The well-documented case of Fanny Albo has become a rallying point for many who oppose such policies.[8] Mrs. Albo, 91, had lived with her 96-year-old husband for over 70 years until a series of medical problems necessitated that they both be hospitalized. Although both were placed initially in the same acute-care facility, Mrs. Albo was deemed eligible for long-term care and was assigned to the first available bed in the region. In this case the bed was more than 100 kilometers away, and the Albos had little opportunity to say goodbye before Mrs. Albo was whisked away in an ambulance. Mrs. Albo died two days later and neither her husband nor her family had an opportunity to say a proper goodbye.

The negative publicity surrounding the Albo case prompted the minister of health in British Columbia to call for a review of the case and the implications of the "First Available Bed" policy.[9] But just as tough cases make bad laws and should not serve as the basis for new policies, typical cases that are poorly or improperly managed should not be the basis for removing a policy that may be otherwise effective. Although the administrators in the Albo case applied the policy according to the letter of the law, they failed to consider relevant particulars of the Albos' situation, including the fact that Mr. Albo was gravely ill and hospital-bound and that the bed to which Mrs. Albo was transferred would make it virtually impossible for the couple to have any contact whatsoever. Although the British Columbia review produced a number of recommendations regarding the need for additional resources and steps to ensure that the policy is employed more effectively and sensitively in the future, there is no recommendation that the "First Available Bed" policy be scrapped and that hospitals revert to the former *laissez-faire* approach.[9]

Despite our best efforts to apply our policy in a fair, equitable, and sensitive manner, situations still arise in which patients and families resist our efforts to move them to the first available bed. We estimate that in about 10%–15% of cases we encounter strong resistance. These cases require extensive consultation, cajoling, and in rare cases even threatened legal action. The stress and distress for all involved is significant. One family refused to complete and sign the application because it simply did not agree with the policy. Family members saw the policy as a violation of their right to choose where their loved one would live and indicated a willingness to pursue the matter in court. In another case family members refused to sign the application because the hospital would not guarantee that their mother would not be sent to a particular home. In this case the woman had a negative experience with this facility many years before and insisted she would never want to go there. After numerous fruitless consultations family members were informed that if they continued to refuse to sign the document the hospital would sign on their behalf. Again this family indicated it was willing to go to court to challenge the hospital's authority. While both of these cases were tremendously stressful, our institution was willing to get a court ruling to settle the legal issue once and for all. However, in both cases the families capitulated at the 11th hour and grudgingly accepted the outcome. Needless to say, the administrative personnel who have had to implement the policy in these tough cases are haunted by the fact that these families at times blame them personally for "ruining our lives."

Outcomes

Our health region encompasses a large geographic area, and in some cases the first available bed could be some distance from the patient's home and family. Our policy addresses this concern directly by acknowledging that the distance of a long-term care facility from the patient's family and support network is an important consideration in deciding whether a particular facility can meet a patient's need. There may be situations when the "first available bed" is not an appropriate bed for a particular patient, as was illustrated so graphically in the Albo case. Hence, at our institution, it is possible that a medically discharged patient will not be transferred to the first available bed in the region if it is judged that the distance from a support network would constitute a greater risk to the patient than the relative lack of physical supports available in acute care. These are judgment calls, of course, and any judgment is influenced or clouded by a variety of subjective factors, leaving it open to question and challenge. But this is the risk we must take as we negotiate the tenuous balance between our organizational need for such a policy and the provision of an appropriate bed for each individual patient.

Clinical ethics consultation generally focuses on individual cases. While it is common to refer to other similar cases in determining an appropriate course of action, each case is unique and must be assessed on its own merits. Many of the contributions to this volume relate experiences with extraordinary cases that have left "moral residue" and accompanying moral distress long after the consultation has taken place.[10] The focus of our discussion was not an individual case but a class of ordinary cases that required an institutional response via a new policy. Policies are developed to respond to institutional needs that are often identified and supported with reference to quantitative data. Such administrative review is necessary and appropriate in any well-managed organization, and it is just such administrative data that generally triggers the process of policy review and development. However, any policy is simply a means to a particular end and should never be treated as an end itself. So while institutional need may trigger the development of a policy in the first place, the individual patient's particular situation must always be considered when the policy is applied. This involves a different role for the ethics consultant.

Despite the trauma associated with transfer to a long-term care facility, the reality is that acute-care beds are at a premium in hospitals across the country, even as the demand for long-term care beds increases. Given this reality, it is our conviction that some version of a "First Available Bed" policy is both practically necessary and ethically defensible. Nevertheless, the fact that patients and their families will continue to experience distress is an indication that both this policy and this process could continue to haunt us for some time, resulting in a different type of "moral residue" than is left by the more typical ethics consultation case.

Discussion questions

1. When if ever is it appropriate to put "organizational needs" ahead of patient needs and/or desires?

2. What would be the moral justification for capitulating to a patient or family request not to transfer to a bed or facility in which the patient would get the most appropriate physical care?
3. Should patients be allowed to stay in an acute-care bed even after they are medically discharged if there is no pressing need for acute-care beds and the community beds available are not in the patient's preferred facility?
4. Are the skills needed for ethics consultation on policy similar to those needed for acute single-case ethics consultation?
5. What are some ways in which a policy can provide flexibility/discretion to address the exceptional case yet limit the potential for abuse and injustice?

REFERENCES

1. Naleppa M. Families and the institutionalized elderly: A review. *J Gerontol Soc Work*, 1996; 27(1/2): 87–111.
2. Dellasega C, Mastrian K. The process and consequences of institutionalizing an elder. *West J Nurs Res*, 1995; 17: 123–40.
3. Melrose S. Reducing relocation stress syndrome in long-term care facilities. *J Practical Nurs*, 2004; 54(4): 15–7.
4. Iwasiw C, Goldenberg D, MacMaster E, McCutcheon S, Bol N. Resident's perspectives on their first two weeks in a long term care facility. *J Clin Nurs*, 1996; 5: 381–8.
5. Mayo NE, Wood-Dauphinee S, Grayton D, Scott SC. Nonmedical bed-days for stroke patients admitted to acute-care hospitals in Montreal, Canada. *Stroke*, 1997; 28: 543–9.
6. Graf C. Functional decline in hospitalized older adults: It's often a consequence of hospitalization, but it doesn't have to be. *Am J Nurs*, 2006; 106(1): 58–67.
7. Wahl J. First available bed discharge policies of Canadian hospitals: Good practice or discrimination on the basis of age and disability? Unpublished manuscript presented at *The Ting Forum on Social Justice: Long-Term Care Stream*. Vancouver, B.C. (October 14, 2006).
8. Changes coming in wake of elderly woman's death. *CBC News*, March 16, 2006. CBC report available at http://www.cbc.ca/canada/british-columbia/story/2006/03/16/bc-fanny-albo20060315.html
9. Penny J. Ballem, MD, FRCP, Deputy Minister of Health BC. *Trail, Seniors Review, Recommendations, March 02, 2006* Ballem Report document available @ http://www.health.gov.bc.ca/cpa/mediasite/pdf/ballem·report.pdf
10. Webster G, Baylis F. Moral residue. In: Rubin SB, Zoloth L, eds. *Margin of Error: The Ethics of Mistakes in the Practice of Medicine*. Hagerstown, MD: University Publishing Group, 2000; 217–32.

Conclusions, educational activities, and references

Denise M. Dudzinski and Paul J. Ford

Concluding comments

Micah Hester, reflecting on the case he presented in this book, eloquently articulates the notion of haunting presented throughout this volume:

> Hauntings can . . . take the form of voices speaking to us, as warnings, as reminders; they can beg and plead. Hauntings are often presented as externally manifest, but they just as often find form as internal, persistent, nagging dialog. Hauntings are typically described as something which is feared, but it seems as plausible to see them as stimulants to reflection and concern, a reminder to be humble and a catalyst for intelligent deliberation.
>
> (Hester, p. 7)

His description encapsulates the variety of ways that authors characterized their haunting cases. In addition to the consultants being haunted, broad conceptual themes tie the cases in this book together. First, every author strives to act with integrity, which requires a combination of being true to oneself and one's profession, adhering to standards and rules, and remaining creative, flexible, and fair. At the beginning of this text, Macauley and Orr initiate the theme of integrity by telling a story of doubt, self-scrutiny, collaboration, forgiveness, and courage. Every subsequent essay implicitly or explicitly addresses personal or professional integrity. Authors describe challenges that a maturing profession should address.[*] Sufficient time has elapsed for full consideration, debate, and incorporation of the American Society for Bioethics and the Humanities' *The Core Competencies in Health Care Ethics Consultation*, guidelines that have become our professional practice standards. The essays in this book demonstrate how these commitments to core standards "play out" in complex cases.

---

[*] While there is debate about whether ethics consultation can properly be called a profession, we use the term to recognize that we have some of the characteristics and certainly the earnestness of a profession.

Because our profession welcomes consultants from an array of disciplines, every consultant, new or seasoned, has much to teach and to learn (see DeMarco & Ford; Swota; Hester; Pinkus, Smetanka & Kottkamp; Bernal; and Agich). Most consultants balance professional responsibilities and the culture of their primary training (medicine, nursing, social work, law, etc.) with those of ethics consultation. Those who wear "two hats" are mindful of responsibilities and expectations in their ethics role, as well as the misperception and confusion that arises while playing multiple roles. Essays by Diekema, Weise, and Chang and Dudzinski explicitly tackle this ubiquitous challenge.

Moral distress looms large in these case studies. It arises when our actions are inconsistent with our beliefs. At times we think we know the right thing to do but feel constrained or powerless to act upon it.[1,2] Ethics consultants assuage the distress of colleagues and patients, as authors Zaner, Spike; Skeel and Williams; Daly and Griggins; Dudzinski; DeMarco and Ford; and Foglia and Pearlman discuss. But because these cases are multifaceted and often tragic, we simultaneously cope with our own moral and emotional distress. While Richard Zaner has taken the lead in writing narratives of the "lived experience" of clinical ethics consultants, we believe more attention to the emotional and haunting facets of consultation will improve the quality of our work. In addition, such storytelling is likely to reduce moral distress, which tends to be overwhelming when one feels isolated and alone. By confessing moments of doubt, ambiguity, inexperience, confusion, and error, we embrace the frailty and tenuousness we feel even as others look to us to frame, name, and clarify issues. This does not diminish the importance of scholarly research, ethical analysis, and clear communication skills that are the foundation of our work. Of course, the vulnerability and well-being of those involved in a consultation are always the priority. But after we have attended to others, we are wise to turn to introspection.

Perhaps the most vexing and pervasive source of anxiety for ethics consultants occurs when clinical issues interface with organizational and social ones. We share the frustration and powerlessness social workers, physicians, nurses, and chaplains suffer when a patient no longer needs acute care and must be discharged, but the only available skilled nursing facility is a dismal place to call home (see essays by Shannon and Pullman *et al.*). What do we have to offer in such consultations? Sometimes it is only after retrospective review that we see the ethical landscape clearly. For example, are we overstepping our bounds to report the resident who made a poor and harmful judgment while moonlighting at another hospital? (See Foglia & Pearlman.) For all of our training in clinical ethics, many of us find that we need more instruction in organizational ethics – in crafting policies, shaping culture, and effecting organizational changes that address the antecedents to recurring ethics consultations. (See essays in "The Big Picture: Organizational Issues.")

Reading these essays with an eye toward quality improvement, several themes stand out. Consultations regarding medical futility and end-of-life decision making continue to draw our attention, but we see more patients with multiple admissions. When patients return, it is not uncommon for the process of conflict resolution to begin anew. (See Ford, and Skeel & Williams.) Opportunities to improve the continuity of our practice can come in many forms. For instance, ethics consultation may be improved by stronger collaborations with psychiatry. In cases where psychiatric and ethical issues are enmeshed the outcomes are haunting for patients, families, and care providers alike. (See essays in "Diversity of desires and limits of liberty: Psychiatric/psychological issues.") Finally, when clinical innovation is involved, we have to quickly gather information about complex medical procedures in order to offer assistance in real time. Without understanding the medical contours, we can misunderstand important elements of the ethical question. Perhaps a "preventive ethics" approach is most effective whereby individuals with ethics training are regularly involved in patient rounds, team meetings, and policy discussions.

We would like to thank the authors for their candor and courage. We hope these cases will enlighten, console, and instruct ethics consultants, members of ethics committees, and bioethics students. We anticipate that these cases will stimulate reflection, humility, and intelligent deliberation in readers. Readers can find solace in knowing other consultants share their tentativeness, doubt, fortitude, resilience, regret, and sadness.

Educational activities overview

This book is a valuable educational resource for ethics consultants, ethics committees, and bioethics students. Below, we outline a variety of ways that the chapters can be used for teaching in multiple contexts, and we provide pedagogical guidance for instructors as well as for learners. *Improving Competence in Clinical Ethics Consultation: A Learner's Guide* (heretofore referred to as "Learner's Guide"), soon to be published by the American Society for Bioethics and the Humanities, complements the activities outlined below and is frequently referenced. In graduate courses, our book can be effectively used in conjunction with a text such as Fletcher et al.'s *Introduction to Clinical Ethics*.

Ethics Committee Education (General)
The following cases reflect a variety of issues faced by ethics committees, address core ethics competencies, or are instructive for improving ethics consultation:

1. Quality of life – and of ethics consultation – in the NICU (R.C. Macauley and R.R. Orr)
2. She was the life of the party (D.S. Diekema)
3. Adolescent pregnancy, confidentiality, and culture (D. Brunnquell)

4. Helping staff help a "hateful" patient: the case of TJ (J.D. Skeel and K.S. Williams)
5. Ulysses contract (B.J. Daly and C. Griggins)
6. Amputate my arm, please. I don't want it anymore (D.M. Dudzinski)
7. You're the ethicist; I'm just the surgeon (J.P. DeMarco and P.J. Ford)
8. One way out: destination therapy by default (A. Chang and D.M. Dudzinski)
9. Listening to the husband (E.W. Bernal)
10. It's not my responsibility (M.B. Foglia and R.A. Pearlman)
11. Intra-operative exposure to sporadic Creutzfeldt-Jakob disease: to disclose or not to disclose (J. Potash)
12. Why do we have to discharge this patient? (S.E. Shannon)
13. Who's that sleeping in my bed? An institutional response to an organizational ethics problem (D. Pullman, R. Singleton, and J. Templeton)

Focused study by theme

In this section, we list chapters that can be used to explore themes beyond those listed in the table of contents.

Legal issues: The following chapters comment on the use or application of law:

1. Quality of life – and of ethics consultation – in the NICU (R.C. Macauley and R.R. Orr)
2. Susie's voice (R.L. Pinkus, S.L. Smetanka, and N.A. Kottkamp)
3. Helping staff help a "hateful" patient: the case of TJ (J.D. Skeel and K.S. Williams)
4. Ulysses contract (B.J. Daly and C. Griggins)
5. Why do we have to discharge this patient? (S.E. Shannon)
6. Who's that sleeping in my bed? An institutional response to an organizational ethics problem (D. Pullman, R. Singleton, and J. Templeton)
7. Intra-operative exposure to sporadic Creutzfeldt-Jakob disease: to disclose or not to disclose (J. Potash)
8. Access to an infant's family: lingering effects of not talking with parents (D.M. Hester)
9. The sound of chains (J. Spike)
10. Adolescent pregnancy, confidentiality, and culture (D. Brunnquell)
11. When a baby dies in pain (T.R. McCormick and D. Woodrum)

Multiple professional roles: The following authors explore the challenges faced in differentiating the special roles and responsibilities in ethics consultation from those of their primary disciplines.

1. Futility, Islam, and death (K.L. Weise)
2. When the patient refuses to eat (D. Craig and G.R. Winslow)

3. She was the life of the party (D.S. Diekema)
4. When a baby dies in pain (T.R. McCormick and D. Woodrum)
5. Altruistic organ donation: Credible? Acceptable? (R.B. Miller)
6. One way out: destination therapy by default (A. Chang and D.M. Dudzinski)

Explicit discussion of models used (individual vs. committee): Three consultation models are generally used. Consultations are performed by a single consultant, a subcommittee, or the full ethics committee. The following chapters highlight the challenges of various models.

1. Quality of life – and of ethics consultation – in the NICU (R.C. Macauley and R.R. Orr)
2. She was the life of the party (D.S. Diekema)
3. When a baby dies in pain (T.R. McCormick and D. Woodrum)
4. Altruistic organ donation: Credible? Acceptable? (R.B. Miller)
5. One way out: destination therapy by default (A. Chang and D.M. Dudzinski)
6. Listening to the husband (E.W. Bernal)
7. Adolescent pregnancy, confidentiality, and culture (D. Brunnquell)
8. It's not my responsibility (M.B. Foglia and R.A. Pearlman)
9. Who's that sleeping in my bed? An institutional response to an organizational ethics problem (D. Pullman, R. Singleton, and J. Templeton)

Impediments to talking directly to patient/family: Generally, firsthand information is sought from patients and families. However, a variety of obstacles can complicate direct communication, as seen in the following cases.

1. Access to an infant's family: lingering effects of not talking with parents (D.M. Hester)
2. It's not my responsibility (M.B. Foglia and R.A. Pearlman)
3. Intra-operative exposure to sporadic Creutzfeldt-Jakob disease: to disclose or not to disclose (J. Potash)
4. Susie's voice (R.L. Pinkus, S.L. Smetanka, and N.A. Kottkamp)
5. Listening to the husband (E.W. Bernal)

Intraprofessional disagreement among consultants/committee members: Disagreements among consultants, while expected, can intensify and complicate the consultation process. The following cases discuss such disagreements.

1. Quality of life – and of ethics consultation – in the NICU (R.C. Macauley and R.R. Orr)
2. Altruistic organ donation: Credible? Acceptable? (R.B. Miller)
3. It's not my responsibility (M.B. Foglia and R.A. Pearlman)

Philosophical approaches to clinical ethics: The following chapters provide comments with stronger philosophical reference.

1. But how *can* we choose? (R.M. Zaner)
2. Maternal–fetal surgery and the "profoundest question in ethics" (M.J. Bliton)

3. Amputate my arm, please. I don't want it anymore (D.M. Dudzinski)
4. Suffering as God's will (K. Ohnsorge and P.J. Ford)

Outpatient challenges: Clinical ethics consultations happen in outpatient settings or stretch over inpatient and outpatient stays. The following cases highlight the special characteristics of consulting under these circumstances.
1. But how *can* we choose? (R.M. Zaner)
2. Maternal–fetal surgery and the "profoundest question in ethics" (M.J. Bliton)
3. Altruistic organ donation: Credible? Acceptable? (R.B. Miller)
4. Adolescent pregnancy, confidentiality, and culture (D. Brunnquell)
5. "Tanya, the one with Jonathan's kidney": a living unrelated donor case of church associates (T.D. Rosell)
6. Susie's voice (R.L. Pinkus, S.L. Smetanka, and N.A. Kottkamp)
7. Who's that sleeping in my bed? An institutional response to an organizational ethics problem (D. Pullman, R. Singleton, and J. Templeton)
8. Intra-operative exposure to sporadic Creutzfeldt-Jakob disease: to disclose or not to disclose (J. Potash)
9. One way out: destination therapy by default (A. Chang and D.M. Dudzinski)

Resource utilization (explicit and implicit): Justice or resource utilization is a common backdrop in ethics consultation, as in the following cases:
1. The sound of chains (J. Spike)
2. Misjudging needs: a messy spiral of complexity (P.J. Ford)
3. Who's that sleeping in my bed? An institutional response to an organizational ethics problem (D. Pullman, R. Singleton, and J. Templeton)
4. Helping staff help a "hateful" patient: the case of TJ (J.D. Skeel and K.S. Williams)

Cross-references by section

Most of the cases in this book can be cross-referenced under multiple section headings. Cases may be listed multiple times.

The most vulnerable of us: pediatrics:
1. Adolescent pregnancy, confidentiality, and culture (D. Brunnquell)
2. Quality of life – and of ethics consultation – in the NICU (R.C. Macauley and R.R. Orr)
3. When a baby dies in pain (T.R. McCormick and D. Woodrum)
4. But how *can* we choose? (R.M. Zaner)
5. Maternal–fetal surgery and the "profoundest question in ethics" (M.J. Bliton)

Diversity of desires and limits of liberty: psychiatric/psychological issues:
1. Intra-operative exposure to sporadic Creutzfeldt-Jakob disease: to disclose or not to disclose (J. Potash)
2. Amputate my arm, please. I don't want it anymore (D.M. Dudzinski)

3. One way out: destination therapy by default (A. Chang and D.M. Dudzinski)
4. Altruistic organ donation: Credible? Acceptable? (R.B. Miller)
5. "Tanya, the one with Jonathan's kidney": a living unrelated donor case of church associates (T.D. Rosell)

Withholding therapy with a twist:
1. Quality of life – and of ethics consultation – in the NICU (R.C. Macauley and R.R. Orr)
2. When a baby dies in pain (T.R. McCormick and D. Woodrum)
3. Access to an infant's family: lingering effects of not talking with parents (D.M. Hester)
4. The sound of chains (J. Spike)
5. She was the life of the party (D.S. Diekema)
6. Susie's voice (R.L. Pinkus, S.L. Smetanka, and N.A. Kottkamp)
7. Feuding surrogates, herbal therapies, and a dying patient (A.H. Swota)
8. One way out: destination therapy by default (A. Chang and D.M. Dudzinski)
9. Misjudging needs: a messy spiral of complexity (P.J. Ford)
10. Why do we have to discharge this patient? (S.E. Shannon)

The unspeakable/unassailable: religious and cultural beliefs:
1. She was the life of the party (D.S. Diekema)
2. Listening to the husband (E.W. Bernal)

Human guinea pigs and miracles: clinical innovation/unorthodox treatments:
1. But how can *we* choose? (R.M. Zaner)
2. Maternal–fetal surgery and the "profoundest question in ethics" (M.J. Bliton)

The big picture: organizational issues:
1. Quality of life – and of ethics consultation – in the NICU (R.C. Macauley and R.R. Orr)
2. Altruistic organ donation: Credible? Acceptable? (R.B. Miller)
3. Misjudging needs: a messy spiral of complexity (P.J. Ford)
4. One way out: destination therapy by default (A. Chang and D.M. Dudzinski)
5. Listening to the husband (E.W. Bernal)

Questions and educational activities for self-study and group activities

Suggested preseminar writing assignments for discussion in seminar:
1. Reflect on a case that haunts you. Why does it haunt you? Does your experience resonate with experiences described by authors in this book? How do you cope with being haunted, and how has it impacted your practice as an ethics consultant?

2. Using any of the cases in the book, write a *chart note* as if you were the consultant. What ethical and professional issues should be identified, defined, and analyzed? Which issues are most important to emphasize? Why?

3. What aspects of your work as an ethics consultant or committee member cause you moral distress? How does your committee help you? What institutional steps can be taken to minimize moral distress for healthcare providers as well as for ethics consultants?

4. "Review your institution's policies on end-of-life care (e.g., limiting life-sustaining treatment, DNR orders, futility, brain death). For each policy, identify five frequently asked questions that clinicians and patients are likely to ask and prepare clear written responses. In a large group or in pairs, review, commend, and make recommendations about each other's responses." (From *Learner's Guide,* "End-of-Life Decision Making.")

For questions 5–30, we suggest having each person write a response and then discuss responses in the larger group.

Conflicts, justice, error, and moral distress:

5. Clarify, define, and distinguish the justice issues that arise in the following cases.
   a. It's not my responsibility (M.B. Foglia and R.A. Pearlman)
   b. Misjudging the needs: a messy spiral of complexity (P.J. Ford)
   c. One way out: destination therapy by default (A. Chang and D.M. Dudzinski)
   d. Who's that sleeping in my bed? An institutional response to an organizational ethics problem (D. Pullman, R. Singleton, and J. Templeton)
   e. The sound of chains (J. Spike)
   f. Ulysses contract (B.J. Daly and C. Griggins)

6. Cases that involve adverse events or errors pose special challenges for ethics consultants. In your experience, what are these challenges and how are they best handled? Compare your experiences with those described in:
   a. Intra-operative exposure to sporadic Creutzfeldt-Jakob disease: to discolse or not to disclose (J. Potash)
   b. Listening to the husband (E.W. Bernal)
   c. It's not my responsibility (M.B. Foglia and R.A. Pearlman)

7. When and how should ethics consultants address the providers' moral distress? Is this a "legitimate" ethics consultation? Why or why not?
   a. Introduction: Live and learn: courage, honesty, and vulnerability (P.J. Ford and D.M. Dudzinski)
   b. Is a broken jaw a terminal condition? (S.G. Finder)
   c. Why do we have to discharge this patient? (S.E. Shannon)
   d. Ulysses contract (B.J. Daly and C. Griggins)
   e. It's not my responsibility (M.B. Foglia and R.A. Pearlman)

8. In the following cases, discuss the sources of conflicts between professional groups and the ways consultants can help address such conflicts.

    a. Is a broken jaw a terminal condition? (S.G. Finder)
    b. It's not my responsibility (M.B. Foglia and R.A. Pearlman)
    c. Intra-operative exposure to sporadic Creutzfeldt-Jakob disease: to disclose or not to disclose (J. Potash)
    d. Why do we have to discharge this patient? (S.E. Shannon)
       (See *Learner's Guide*, "Negotiating difference and accounting for context.")

Surrogate decision making:

9. Compare two of the following cases and discuss the conditions under which a surrogate's decision should and should not be challenged.
    a. When a baby dies in pain (T.R. McCormick and D. Woodrum)
    b. Why do we have to discharge this patient? (S.E. Shannon)
    c. The sound of chains (J. Spike)
    d. When the patient refuses to eat (D. Craig and G.R. Winslow)
    e. Is a broken jaw a terminal condition? (S.G. Finder)
    f. Feuding surrogates, herbal therapies, and a dying patient (A.H. Swota)
       (See *Learner's Guide*, "Surrogate Decision-Making".)
10. Discuss and compare the following decision-making capacity cases:
    a. Helping staff help a "hateful" patient: the case of TJ (J.D. Skeel and K.S. Williams)
    b. Suffering as God's will (K. Ohnsorge and P.J. Ford)
    c. Altruistic organ donation: Credible? Acceptable? (R.B. Miller)
       (See *Learner's Guide*, "Decision-making capacity.")

Autonomy and its limits:

11. When and why are we justified in questioning or overriding the autonomous wishes of competent patients? Compare the following cases:
    a. Ulysses contract (B.J. Daly and C. Griggins)
    b. Amputate my arm, please. I don't want it anymore (D.M. Dudzinski)
12. How should consultants help negotiate the conflict between a patient's choice and the provider's professional obligations?
    a. Amputate my arm, please. I don't want it anymore (D.M. Dudzinski)
    b. Ulysses contract (B.J. Daly and C. Griggins)
    c. Altruistic kidney donation: Credible? Acceptable? (R.B. Miller)
    d. "Tanya, the one with Jonathan's kidney": a living unrelated donor case of church associates (T.D. Rosell)

Roles, process, and perception of ethics consultation:

13. How does your committee or consultation service avoid being seen as the "ethics police" while still maintaining courage to challenge authorities? Compare the responses of consultants in the following cases with your own examples. Scrutinize the factors that prompt you to challenge or *not* challenge authority.

a. Intra-operative exposure to sporadic Creutzfeldt-Jakob disease: to disclose or not to disclose (J. Potash)

b. It's not my responsibility (M.B. Foglia and R.A. Pearlman)

c. Misjudging needs: a messy spiral of complexity (P. Ford)

14. Using any of the cases in the book, envision several ways the consultant may have been perceived by a patient, family, attending physician, nurse, or clinician who objected to the ethics consultation.

15. Compare the "lived experience" of being a new consultant or consultant in training with the experience of a seasoned, confident ethics consultant. What are the affective and cognitive advantages and disadvantages of each role?

a. Listening to the husband (E.W. Bernal)

b. Access to an infant's family: lingering effects of not talking with parents (D.M. Hester)

c. You're the ethicist; I'm just the surgeon (J.P. DeMarco and P.J. Ford)

d. Haunted by a good outcome: the case of Sister Jane (G.J. Agich)

e. The sound of chains (J. Spike)

f. Is a broken jaw a terminal condition? (S.G. Finder)

16. Discuss whether and how ethics consultants should question, verify, or challenge the clinical judgments of those requesting a consultation or of those treating the patient.

a. Suffering as God's will (K. Ohnsorge and P.J. Ford)

b. Haunted by a good outcome: the case of Sister Jane (G.J. Agich)

c. When the patient refuses to eat (D. Craig and G.R. Winslow)

17. In an ethics consultation, what type of patient information should (and should not) be gathered? Once gathered in the consultation process, with whom should information be shared (family members, ethicists outside the institution, general counsel)? Do we need a patient's permission to review a chart or share information with colleagues? How does the Health Insurance Portability and Accountability Act (HIPAA) and institutional policy apply to patient privacy and confidentiality in ethics consultation? Are there other privacy considerations in conducting ethics consultation?

a. Haunted by a good outcome: the case of Sister Jane (G.J. Agich)

b. Misjudging needs: a messy spiral of complexity (P.J. Ford)
(See *Learner's Guide*, "Privacy and Confidentiality.")

18. How do you decide which voices are most important to hear and what strategies should be used to be sure those voices have a proper influence on the clinical decision?

a. Access to an infant's family: lingering effects of not talking with parents (D.M. Hester)

b. Amputate my arm, please. I don't want it anymore (D.M. Dudzinski)

c. Susie's voice (R.L. Pinkus, S.L. Smetanka, and N.A. Kottkamp)
(See *Learner's Guide*, "Negotiating Difference and Accounting for Context.")

19. How do you address professional disagreements among ethics consultants? How do you decide whose opinion should prevail when two consultants have opposing opinions?
20. What, if any, obligation do consultants have when their advice is not taken?
    a. When a baby dies in pain (T.R. McCormick and D. Woodrum)
    b. Listening to the husband (E.W. Bernal)
    c. Intra-operative exposure to sporadic Creutzfeldt-Jakob disease: to disclose or not to disclose (J. Potash)
    d. "Tanya, the one with Jonathan's kidney": a living unrelated donor case of church associates (T.D. Rosell)

Maternal-fetal, perinatal, and pediatric issues:
21. Discuss the special characteristics of maternal-fetal decision making, in which the autonomy and preferences of the woman are balanced with the uncertain prognosis for the fetus.
    a. But how *can* we choose? (R.M. Zaner)
    b. Maternal-fetal surgery and the "profoundest question in ethics" (M.J. Bliton)
22. Describe the framework for decision making in the neonatal intensive care unit (NICU) and pediatric intensive care unit (PICU). Discuss how the culture of neonatal and pediatric medicine impacts ethics consultation.
    a. When a baby dies in pain (T.R. McCormick and D. Woodrum)
    b. The sound of chains (J. Spike)
    c. Access to an infant's family: lingering effects of not talking with parents (D.M. Hester)
    d. Quality of life – and of ethics consultation – in the NICU (R.C. Macauley and R.R. Orr)
    (See *Learner's Guide*, "Ethical Issues Involving Newborns and Critically Ill Infants and Children.")

"Difficult" patients and families:
23. How can we help providers care for "difficult" patients/families such that we both honor the challenges they face and encourage receptiveness to the patient/family and minimization of bias?
    a. Helping staff help a "hateful" patient: the case of TJ (J.D. Skeel and K.S. Williams)
    b. The sound of chains (J. Spike)
    c. Ulysses contract (B.J. Daly and C. Griggins)
    d. When the patient refuses to eat (D. Craig and G.R. Winslow)
    e. Misjudging the needs: a messy spiral of complexity (P.J. Ford)
    f. Futility, Islam, and death (K.L. Weise)
    g. One way out: destination therapy by default (A. Chang and D.M. Dudzinski)

24. Make a list of terms used to describe "difficult" patients. Analyze the judgments, values, and assumptions embedded in these terms. What factors put patients and family members at risk of being labeled "difficult" or "noncompliant"? (From *Learner's Guide*, "Dealing with 'Difficult' Patients: Professional and Institutional Responses.")

Cultural issues:

25. Consider how the "culture of medicine" might look from the points of view of patients and families in the following stories.
    a. Adolescent pregnancy, confidentiality, and culture (D. Brunnquell)
    b. "Tanya, the one with Jonathan's kidney": a living unrelated donor case of church associates (T.D. Rosell)
    c. Futility, Islam, and death (K.L. Weise)
    d. Suffering as God's will (K. Ohnsorge and P.J. Ford)
    e. Susie's voice (R.L. Pinkus, S.L. Smetanka, and N.A. Kottkamp)
26. Compare Swota's "Feuding surrogates, herbal therapies, and a dying patient" with your own cases that involve the use of integrative, traditional, or alternative medicine.

End-of-life issues:

27. Discuss the challenges involved in "medical futility" cases. How do your hospital, local, or state policies impact the handling of these cases? How do you ensure that intractable conflicts are fairly handled, especially when unilateral decisions to override a patient/family's wishes are institutionally sanctioned? How does handling of these cases differ when it is the patient or family who believes continued treatment is unbeneficial (i.e., futile)?
    a. Susie's voice (R.L. Pinkus, S.L. Smetanka, and N.A. Kottkamp)
    b. Misjudging needs: a messy spiral of complexity (P.J. Ford)
    c. You're the ethicist; I'm just the surgeon (J.P. DeMarco and P.J. Ford)
    d. Is a broken jaw a terminal condition? (S.G. Finder)
    e. Futility, Islam, and death (K.L. Weise)
    f. Quality of life – and of ethics consultation – in the NICU (R.C. Macauley and R.R. Orr)
    g. She was the life of the party (D.S. Diekema)
28. How are the issues in "When the patient refuses to eat" by D. Craig and G.R. Winslow similar to and different from typical discussions of withholding artificial nutrition and hydration from adults? From children? Highlight important clinical, ethical, and professional factors that make these types of cases distinct.

Ethics retreats and seminar activities

The cases in this book can be used as a springboard for various types of educational activities. In addition to those listed under "Questions and Educational Activities for Self-Study and Group Activities," activities listed below can be instructive for retreats and longer seminars.

Simulate a case consultation:

1. Use a simulation model to enact one of the cases in the book. Assign consultants to play the part of each major stakeholder and have one person play the ethics consultant. The person playing the ethics consultant conducts a family meeting with the goals of (a) making sure everyone has the opportunity to be heard, (b) identifying sources of conflict, confusion, and disagreement, (c) defining the ethical issues, and (d) facilitating discussion and conflict resolution. Commend the person playing the role of consultant and make recommendations for improving practice. Feedback can be both verbal and in writing. Have each member of the ethics consultation service play the role of ethics consultant and receive feedback. After this exercise, identify the special strengths each consultant brings to the practice. Keep these strengths in mind when you collaborate (either formally or informally) to provide ethics consultation.

   a. For a template of questions to use in providing feedback, see Loyola University's Neiswanger Institute for Bioethics & Health Policy website at http://www.bioethics.lumc.edu. By navigating through the ethics consultation link, you can access the "Skill Building Materials in Case Consultation."

   b. See *Learner's Guide*, "Process Skills in Performing Ethics Case Consultation."

2. At the conclusion of the role-play, all consultants write a chart note. Discuss essential features of the chart note and collect quotes that are particularly succinct and effective in explaining the ethical issues.

Quality improvement:

3. "Review the chart of a patient who received an ethics consultation to find medical, nursing, social, and spiritual/pastoral care information pertinent to the ethics consultation."

   (From *Learner's Guide*, "Information Gathering and Assessment.")

4. Several publications include checklists of questions that should be addressed during an ethics consultation. (See J. C. Fletcher, R. Boyle, *Introduction to Clinical Ethics* [Second Edition], pp. 23–4; A.R. Jonsen, M. Siegler, W. Sinslade, *Clinical Ethics* [6th Edition]; or the *Ethics Consultation Primer* available through the Department of Veterans Affairs National Center for Ethics website at www.va.gov/integratedethics.) Using one of these checklists, read a case from the book to see which questions are and are not addressed in the write-up. How would you find answers to questions that are not addressed? Describe why some questions may not be pertinent in the particular case.

   (See *Learner's Guide*, "Information Gathering and Assessment.")

5. Have an experienced ethics consultant and a new consultant review one of the cases in the book. Have both write chart notes. Debrief together about why certain issues were highlighted by each consultant. Recognize that both new and seasoned consultants have special insights. Notice the differences resulting from diverse disciplinary backgrounds.

6. Review a case in the book and identify two to three ethically acceptable options. Provide rationale and references for why these options would be permissible. Identify one ethically unacceptable option. Provide rationale and references for why this option would be unacceptable.
   (See *Learner's Guide*, "Information Gathering and Assessment.")

7. Have each participant draft a three- to four-sentence description of ethics consultation that can be used when meeting healthcare providers, patients, and families. Compare the scripts in order to draft an introduction that can be used by everyone. Share this script with new consultants.
   (See *Learner's Guide*, "Process Skills in Performing Consultation.")

8. Review several cases in this book and/or chart notes from ethics consultations. Categorize the ethical issues addressed (e.g., confidentiality, decision-making capacity, medical futility). See if all participants agree with the categorizations. Notice if issues are treated similarly in all cases (e.g., Are medical futility cases approached similarly? If not, why not?).

9. Identify hospital, state, and federal policies with which all consultants must be familiar. Using a case from the book, identify which policies and laws are pertinent to the case. If such a case arose at your institution, would it be handled differently based on your policies? Are these policies ethically sound?

10. Review the mediation techniques outlined in *Bioethics Mediation* by N. Dubler and C. Leibman. Apply them to one of the cases in this book. How does mediation differ from consultation? Does mediation enhance or improve ethics consultation? Why or why not?
    (See *Learner's Guide*, "Facilitate Communication and Identify Ethically Acceptable Resolutions.")

11. Discuss the indicators for when an ethics consultation is closed (e.g., chart note written, "signed off"). When is follow-up warranted and when is follow-up beyond the scope and responsibility of "ethics"? Is it permissible to access the patient's record after the case is closed? Why or why not?
    a. Misjudging the needs (P.J. Ford)
    b. Is a broken jaw a terminal condition? (S.G. Finder)

12. Discuss what educational and institutional follow-up you would propose in any of the cases in the section entitled, "The Big Picture: Organizational Issues." What responsibilities do ethics consultants have to change institutional culture and expectations? Provide examples of how the ethics committee or consultation service has impacted the organization and identify institutional issues where ethics should be more involved.

13. "Develop a short 'customer satisfaction' survey for ethics case consultation." Consider distributing to staff after a consultation.
(From *Learner's Guide*, "Feedback and Quality Assurance.")

14. "Write a brief description of your primary role in the institution, specifically the tools, practices, authority, and character associated with the role. Compare and contrast your primary role to that of ethics consultation."
(From *Learner's Guide*, "Responsibilities of Those Engaged in Ethics Consultation.")

15. Discuss ways in which ethics consultants can abuse their power. What steps can you take to avoid misuse of power?
(See *Learner's Guide*, "Responsibilities of Those Engaged in Ethics Consultation.")

16. "Describe the distinctions between moral uncertainty, moral dilemmas, moral distress, and moral residue, and identify positive and negative aspects of the notion of 'moral compromise.'"
(From *Learner's Guide*, "Challenges of the Role: The Experience of Providing Ethics Consultation.")

REFERENCES

Ethics consultation professional practice guidelines

1. Society for Health & Human Values – Society for Bioethics Consultation, Task Force on Standards for Bioethics Consultation. *Core Competencies in Health Care Ethics Consultation: The Report of the American Society for Bioethics and the Humanities.* Glenview, IL: American Society for Bioethics & Humanities, 1998. The core competencies outline the knowledge, attitudes, skills, and character traits essential for competent ethics consultation. This is the professional practice guideline for healthcare ethics consultation.

Educational resource recommended as companion to this book

1. Aulisio MP *et al.*, American Society for Bioethics and Humanities (ASBH) Clinical Ethics Task Force. *Improving Competence in Clinical Ethics Consultation: A Learner's Guide.* American Society for Bioethics and Humanities, 2008. Available at www.asbh.org. The *Learner's Guide* provides an overview of key issues in clinical ethics, along with educational activities and references. The resources and activities recommended are especially suitable for ethics committees and consultation services. A curriculum can be created by integrating the *Learner's Guide*, this book, and the *Core Competencies.*

Selected books and manuscripts

1. Arras JD, Steinbock, B, eds. *Ethical Issues in Modern Medicine*, 5th ed. Mountain View, CA: Mayfield, 1999.
2. Aulisio MP, Arnold RM, Youngner SJ, eds. *Ethics Consultation: From Theory to Practice.* Baltimore, MD: The Johns Hopkins University Press, 2003.

3. Boyle PJ, DuBose ER, Ellingson SJ, Guinn DE, McCurdy DB. *Organizational Ethics in Health Care: Principles, Cases, & Practical Solutions*. San Francisco: Jossey-Bass, 2001.

4. Ashcroft RE, Lucassen A, Parker M, Verkerk M, Widershoven G. *Case Analysis in Clinical Ethics*. New York: Cambridge University Press, 2005.

5. Charon R, Montello M. *Stories Matter: The Role of Narrative in Medical Ethics*. New York: Routledge, 2002.

6. Dickenson DL, Fulford B, Murray T, eds. *Healthcare Ethics and Human Values: An Introductory Text with Readings and Case Studies*. Malden, MA: Blackwell, 2002.

7. Dubler NN, Liebman CB. *Bioethics Mediation: A Guide to Shaping Shared Solutions*. New York: United Hospital Fund of New York, 2004.

8. Fletcher JS, Boyle R. *Introduction to Clinical Ethics*, 3rd ed. Frederick, MD: University Publishing Group, 2005.

9. Hester DM. Ethics by Committee: *A Textbook on Consultation, Organization, and Education for Hospital Ethics Committees*. Lanham, MD: Rowman & Littlefield, 2007.

10. Jecker NS, Jonsen AR, Pearlman RA. *Bioethics: An Introduction to the History, Methods, & Practice*, 2nd ed. Sudbury, MA: Jones and Bartlett, 2007.

11. Jonsen AR, Siegler M, Winslade WJ. *Clinical Ethics: A Practical Approach to Ethical Decisions in Medicine*, 6th ed. New York: McGraw-Hill, 2006.

12. Kuczewski MG, Pinkus RLB. *An Ethics Casebook for Hospitals: Practical Approaches to Everyday Cases*. Washington, DC: Georgetown University Press, 1999.

13. Kushner TK, Thomasma DC, eds. *Ward Ethics: Dilemmas for Medical Students and Doctors in Training*. Cambridge: Cambridge University Press, 2001.

14. Munson R. *Outcomes Uncertain – Cases and Contexts in Bioethics*. Boston, MA: Wadsworth, 2003.

15. Pence G. *Classic Cases in Medical Ethics*, 4th ed. New York: McGraw-Hill, 2004.

16. Post L, Blustein J, Dubler NN. *Handbook for Health Care Committees*. Baltimore, MD: Johns Hopkins University Press, 2007.

17. Redman BK. *Measurement Instruments in Clinical Ethics*. Thousand Oaks, CA: Sage, 2002.

18. Rubin SB, Zoloth L. *Margin of Error: The Ethics of Mistakes in the Practice of Medicine*. Hagerstown, MD: University Publishing Group, 2000.

19. Steinbock B. *The Oxford Handbook of Bioethics*. New York: Oxford University Press, 2007.

20. Tan-Alora A, Lumintao JM. *Beyond a Western Bioethics: Voices from the Developing World*. Washington, DC: Georgetown University Press, 2001.

21. Zaner RM. *Conversations on the Edge: Narratives of Ethics and Illness*. Washington, DC: Georgetown University Press, 2004.

22. Zaner RM. *Ethics and the Clinical Encounter*. Englewood Cliffs, NJ: Prentice Hall, 1998.

23. Zaner RM, ed. *Performance, Talk, Reflection: What Is Going on in Clinical Ethics Consultation?* New York: Springer, 1999.

Bioethics encyclopedia

1. Post SG, ed. *Encyclopedia of Bioethics*, 3rd ed. New York: Macmillan Reference USA, 2003.

Selected ethics websites

1. **www.bioethics.net.** This site culls bioethics-related news, provides introductory information on bioethics topics, maintains a blog, and provides relevant ethics links. It is also the host cite for *The American Journal of Bioethics*.
2. **http://www.ethics.va.gov/ETHICS/activities/integratedethics.asp.** The U.S. Department of Veterans Affairs has developed publicly available resources pertaining to clinical and organizational ethics. Their Integrated Ethics Program includes primers and tools for ethics consultation, preventive ethics, and ethical leadership.
3. **www.asbh.org.** The American Society for Bioethics and the Humanities (ASBH) website. This is the professional association for bioethicists in the United States. Information about regional and annual meetings and ASBH publications are available here.
4. **www.bioethics.ca/index-ang.html.** Canadian Bioethics Society/Société Canádienne de Bioéthique. This is the professional association for Canadian bioethicists. Information about scholarly meetings is available here.
5. **http://bioethics.od.nih.gov.** Bioethics resources compiled by the National Institutes of Health related to education, research involving human subjects, research involving animals, medical and healthcare ethics, applied genetics, and biotechnology.
6. **http://www.ama-assn.org/ama/pub/category/3040.html.** The American Medical Association publishes articles on health law, policy, professionalism, and research. Case studies are available through "The Virtual Mentor" site at the link above.

Selected bioethics journals

For descriptions of bioethics journals, visit www.asbh.org.

a. *Journal of Clinical Ethics*
b. *Hastings Center Report*
c. *American Journal of Bioethics*
d. *Cambridge Quarterly for Health Care Ethics*
e. *Theoretical Medicine and Bioethics*
f. *Journal of Medical Ethics*
g. *Journal of Law, Medicine, and Ethics*
h. *The Kennedy Institute of Ethics Journal*
i. *The Journal of Medicine and Philosophy*
j. *HEC Forum*

Chapter references

1. Jameton A. *Nursing Practice: Ethical Issues*. Englewood Cliffs, NJ: Prentice Hall, 1984.
2. Hardingham L. Integrity and moral residue: Nurses as participants in a moral community. *Nurs Philos*, 2004; 5(2): 127–34.

Index